Optimal Healing

A Guide to Traditional Chinese Medicine

Patricia Tsang, M.D.

Balance for Health Publishing

Balance for Health Publishing
3701 Sacramento St. #407
San Francisco, CA 94118

www.balanceforhealthpublishing.com

The material set forth in this book is for informational and educational pur-poses. It should not be construed to constitute medical advice or to replace consultation with a qualified healthcare provider for diagnosis and treatment of illness or disease.

Publisher's Cataloging-in-Publication
(Provided by Quality Books, Inc.)

Tsang, Patricia.
    Optimal healing : a guide to traditional Chinese
    medicine / Patricia Tsang. — 1st ed.
    p. cm.
    Includes bibliographical references and index.

    1. Medicine, Chinese.   I. Title.

    R601.T73 2007   610'.951
                             QBI07-600235

Book cover and interior design by 1106 Design
Illustrations by Jennifer Suehs

ISBN: 978-0-9799484-9-7

Library of Congress Control Number: 2007907373

To my teacher,

Yat Ki Lai, L.Ac., O.M.D.

"Dr. Tsang has done an outstanding job of interpreting the ancient practice of TCM into contemporary Western medical terms. She does this in a very accessible and engaging manner, weaving in case examples that bring the practice of TCM alive."

Priscilla Abercrombie, RN, NP, PhD, Assistant Clinical Professor
UCSF Department of Ob/Gyn and Reproductive Science and
Community Health Systems Nursing

"A superb overview that will enable patients, students, and health professionals to better understand Traditional Chinese Medicine and its integration into Western medical practice. The book is lucid and engaging, filled with personal examples that draw in the reader and help clarify the often strange-sounding TCM terms, while providing specific information on diagnosis and therapy. The author is a Western trained physician who later learned TCM and integrated it into her practice, way before it became as fashionable as it now is. I think this would be a terrific book for every new student of acupuncture and Oriental medicine to read as they begin and then continue their studies."

Gary M Arsham, MD, PhD
Chair, California Pacific Medical Center Institutional Review Board
Member of Advisory Board, Seattle Institute of Oriental Medicine
Co-author of *Diabetes: A guide to Living Well* and *101 Tips for Coping with Diabetes*

"In *Optimal Healing,* Patricia Tsang offers an informed exploration of traditional Chinese medicine (TCM) and its interface with Western biomedicine. She writes as a board-certified anesthesiologist who has also made an intensive study of TCM. The book is filled with acute clinical observations, scientific findings, and probing analysis of the research opportunities in TCM that would greatly expand our understanding of human healing."

Michael Lerner, PhD, president, Commonweal
Author of *Choices in Healing: The Best of Conventional and Complementary Approaches to Cancer*

"From reading this marvelous book, written by a physician trained in both Western and Eastern medicine, I have gained a basic understanding of herbal and acupuncture treatments. With this new knowledge, I can now better relate to my patients who have been successfully treated with complementary approaches. I also found the section on foods and diet enlightening. I recommend it for every practicing physician as well as every medical student."

Cynthia Point, M.D. internist, San Francisco, AOA,
member ACP, Best Doctor category Internist 2000, 2002–2007

"This is a landmark book that bridges the gap between Eastern and Western medicine. It truly demystifies traditional Chinese medicine. I appreciate how the author has set straight that there are stages to disease and a best time to use Eastern versus Western medicine."

Derrina Wu, M.D., internist
San Francisco

Contents

Preface

The first five chapters of this book are devoted to translating the mystical-sounding terms used in traditional Chinese medicine into familiar contemporary language. I take you into the classroom at the American College of Traditional Chinese Medicine as I listen to the lectures and ponder their meaning. The lecturer's words are italicized. The lectures were delivered in Cantonese by Ken Pang, L.Ac. and translated into English by Sifu Fong Ha, a martial arts master. The material was compiled from both ancient classic literature and contemporary traditional Chinese medical books.

In traditional Chinese medicine (TCM), organs often represent several physiologic systems rather than the organs as we know them. Whenever used in the TCM sense, these organs, mainly the Liver, Kidney, and Spleen, have been capitalized to distinguish them from the organs we know as the liver, kidney, and spleen.

Causes of disease in TCM are classified according to the six evils: Cold, Fire, Summer Heat, Dryness, Wetness, and Wind. These terms likewise are capitalized when used in the TCM sense. TCM conditions, or symptom patterns, are classified according to the eight entities: Yin, Yang, Hot, Cold, Internal, External, Solid, and

Deficient. They represent four pairs of dualities and, when used in this context, are also capitalized.

Terms in Chinese can have several English translations. "Liver Fire uprising" can also be called "Liver Fire," "Deficiency Fire," or "Insubstantial Heat." Regarding the Six Evils, Dryness is sometimes called Parchness; Wet is sometimes translated as Damp. Regarding the eight entities, "Deficiency" is also known as "Vacuity." The term "Mobilizing Qi and Blood" is interchangeable with "Vitalizing Qi and Blood."

From the sixth chapter on, after having explained the meaning of TCM terms, I go on to explain the TCM paradigm, point out how it differs from the Western paradigm, and demonstrate its relevance in my contemporary integrated practice. The case studies are all true, but the patients' names have been changed to protect privacy.

Introduction

One day, after I performed acupuncture on a new patient, she told me, "I'm disappointed. I expected your office to have beaded curtains and more of an Asian aura. Your treatment room is just like any other doctor's office." The Western stereotype of Chinese medicine dies hard. The media tend to cover stories about acupuncture by focusing on its mystical appeal. In television segments the camera is pointed at patients with needles protruding from their faces. Exotic music plays in the background. A practitioner pronounces an incantation that no one, possibly not even he himself, understands: "The problem is that your Qi is obstructed."

While the romantic in us is drawn to magic shows and the like, if we perpetuate a romanticized view of traditional Chinese medicine (TCM), we forfeit a multitude of benefits. But if we strive to understand this ancient system of healing, we can learn about disease prevention, find ways to resolve many chronic intractable conditions, and contain health-care cost. The purpose of this book is to demystify TCM by translating its terms into familiar language, explain its unique paradigm, dispel some common misconceptions about it, and recommend ways in which it can be used to complement Western medicine.

Many of the mystical-sounding terms used by traditional Chinese practitioners actually have concrete meanings. The terms sound strange because they are over three thousand years old, originating at a time when there was little knowledge of anatomy, physiology, or microbiology. Each term, though, represents some physiological phenomenon. As a Western-trained physician who experienced healing from an intractable condition using Chinese herbs, I became interested in TCM, studied it, and actually put this system to use in my practice of family medicine. By doing this, I have been able to help many patients whose conditions were considered hopeless. My explanations cannot be found in any existing reference books. They are the result of my studying English translations of the ancient Chinese texts, wrapping my Western-trained mind around the odd-sounding terms and concepts, finding Western equivalents for them, and ultimately applying the teachings to treating patients.

No one can deny that we have benefited enormously from the advances made by Western medicine. Neither can we deny that Western medicine is facing some serious problems. With the discovery of antibiotics and vaccines, people are living longer. Now the challenge has partially shifted from fighting common infectious diseases to treating degenerative diseases and cancer. Yet with our overuse and misuse of antibiotics, an even greater threat has emerged: the growing number of drug-resistant microorganisms, which drives the need for constant research and development of new drugs. Elaborate and increasingly expensive tests are prerequisites for diagnosis and treatment in the Western medical paradigm. Our treatments are mostly directed at late, advanced stages of disease, but we have few options for the early stages of disease. All these problems are fueling the skyrocketing cost of health care.

Healing depends on both interventional treatment to fight disease and the patient's own bodily ability to heal itself. The

Western approach ignores the latter part of this equation. Early in the HIV-AIDS epidemic, we should have learned that no matter how many smart bombs we use to target infectious organisms, if the patient's immune system has been ravaged, recovery is unlikely. Eastern medicine directs attention not only toward fighting the disease but also toward strengthening the weakened bodily mechanism of the host in order to promote self-healing. Both Eastern and Western medicine have inherent strengths and weaknesses. Thus, integration of both paradigms can promote optimal health care.

While Westerners have developed a fascination with Eastern medicine, their approach to employing the system is misdirected. To isolate the active ingredients of herbs in order to use them for fighting disease is a Western concept. In Eastern medicine, herbs to fight disease are used in combination with herbs to strengthen the patient. Missing this important duality may lead to failure in our quest for holistic medicine.

The other flaw in the Western approach to using Eastern treatments is inappropriate timing. At present, the Western medical establishment turns to "alternative" Eastern treatments as a last resort after all Western methods have been exhausted. Eastern treatments, aimed at normalizing the host's own healing mechanisms, should logically be used in the early stages of disease when there is a better chance for reversal.

For seventeen years, I used an integration of Eastern and Western medicine to treat many patients in the competitive arena of private practice in San Francisco, where there is a doctor glut. When pre-paid insurance plans, Health Maintenance Organizations (HMOs), became prevalent, my medical practice underwent the usual HMO cost scrutiny. It proved to be one of the most cost-effective primary care practices in my area. I attribute this success to my knowing when and how to use traditional Chinese treatments appropriately. For viral respiratory infections, I prescribed herbal treatments, and most of my patients recovered quickly without developing bronchitis and without requiring antibiotics. Integrating herbs into my treatment regime for asthmatics prevented many emergency room visits. For musculoskeletal problems, I used acupuncture and ordered fewer expensive imaging tests such as MRIs. When patients felt better after the treatments, those tests became unnecessary. I also prescribed fewer nonsteroidal anti-inflammatory drugs, and, as a result, my patients suffered fewer drug reactions. Integrating traditional Chinese medicine into my practice has enabled me to better adhere to the dictum "First, do no harm," and to contain health-care costs.

To my readers, whether patient or healer, I want to bring hope and awareness that if you have reached an impasse with using the conventional Western approach, there is a whole other approach worth exploring.

Chapter 1

Beginnings

It all began in the third year of my Western medical school training. For the class of '63 at the University of California San Francisco School of Medicine, it was a time of extremes. First was the heady realization that we had at last ascended to the elite status of being called doctor, let loose on the unsuspecting patients of San Francisco General Hospital (SF General). Could they tell that we were not really truly doctors yet? Our practicum was about to begin. One of my classmates paraded around town in his newly acquired white lab coat. He began to have second thoughts about such ostentation when someone in a public parking lot asked him to park his car. The final blow to his ego came at the supermarket when someone asked him, "Where is the aisle for canned soup?" Later came our descent into hopeless hypochondria. We imagined we had every disease described in every medical textbook we read. Going through dermatology rotation, most of us imagined every mole we had was a malignant melanoma. Medical students requesting biopsies overran the skin clinic.

One day, while rotating through the pediatrics service at San Francisco General Hospital, I felt ill. (Back then, the pediatrics ward was equivalent to today's day-care center in terms of being the most efficient propagator of infectious diseases known to man.) I experienced chills, fever, and a cough. My brother Wally, then an intern at Santa Clara County and two years ahead of me, diagnosed pneumonia over the phone. My professor of internal medicine confirmed Wally's diagnosis. He promptly put me in the hospital and prescribed antibiotics. After a week, I was much improved. Soon I was allowed to return to classes and the work of seeing patients at SF General. I felt well except for one thing—a persistent, dry, hacking cough, usually worse in the evening. The prescribed cough medicine with codeine only made me nauseated without relieving the cough. Patients teased me that I sounded as if I needed a doctor more than they did. This went on for over a month. Thoughts of saving the ills of the world soon faded as I struggled to get myself better.

My mother ultimately came to my rescue. Mom believed in Western medicine and followed doctors' orders assiduously. She was one of those who would set her alarm clock to take her pill on time if it was prescribed every six hours. Yet when Western medicine had been tried and failed, she was not above turning to Chinese remedies. She consulted with one of her friends about my cough. Mom's friend recommended that I see a well-known Chinese herbalist, Dr. Ding Jung-Ying. Out of desperation, I agreed to do so. Dr. Ding's office was located in the heart of San Francisco Chinatown, up several flights of stairs. Unlike my family doctor's office, Dr. Ding's was sparsely furnished with only a small writing table and several chairs. Looking around, I saw none of the medical equipment usual in a doctor's office. Dr. Ding was elderly and spoke only Chinese. Correctly assuming that my Chinese would be inadequate, he directed his questions about my illness to my mother. He then felt my radial pulse in each wrist, looked at my tongue, wrote a prescription in Chinese, and gave my mother instructions about brewing the herbs he had prescribed. It was not an unpleasant experience for me. No tongue depressor to look into my throat, which always caused me to gag, no cold stethoscope on my chest, and best of all, no shots. I timidly clung to the hope that his remedy would work. We paid the doctor, and my mother and I went off to fill the prescription at an herbal store in Chinatown. Cooking the herbs filled the kitchen with a familiar pungent odor of yesteryear when Mom would coax me to drink similar awful concoctions for colds and the flu. After taking two doses of the nasty stuff, my cough disappeared. It never returned.

I was both impressed and elated. Memories returned of my brother Don's experience when he was in his teens. Mom had taken him to see an herbalist for pain in his knees, which, in retrospect, were most likely growing pains. Upon his return from the visit, Don described to us with great excitement how the Chinese doctor was able to tell from just feeling his pulses that he had had malaria as a young boy. I also thought of our family physician and friend who told us about his experience as a medical student. While doing autopsies one hot summer in Chicago, he contracted a disease that defied diagnosis by his professors. Finally, in a scenario similar to mine, his parents took him to a Chinese herbalist whose remedies eliminated his symptoms.

If ever the opportunity arose, I decided, I would study Traditional Chinese Medicine (TCM). The problem, though, was that my Chinese literacy was probably below first grade level. I grew up in San Francisco. My parents, fluent in both English and Cantonese Chinese, required that I attend Chinese school after elementary school. Chinese school was the bane of every Chinese American schoolchild's existence. While our American classmates played after regular school, we had to continue with more classes. When I turned twelve, I was released from that requirement. With disuse, I quickly forgot most of what I learned about written Chinese. My biggest regret is not being able to read a menu in Chinese restaurants. The Chinese version often offers an assortment of bargain dishes not in the English version, and the waiter treats you with a bit more deference if you know written Chinese. In the 1960s there were no schools in the United States teaching TCM in English, so my idea of learning it was more a dream than a real possibility. Nineteen years passed before my dream came to fruition. Meanwhile, I had trained in anesthesiology and intensive care. I had gone to Taiwan to do some work for a Christian clinic. Upon my return, I carved out a career in emergency medicine where my anesthesiology training proved very useful.

In 1980, my Aunt Teresa came to visit us from Macao. Whereas my father was a reserved man with a subtle wit, his younger siblings could be considered flamboyant. Dad's sister, Teresa, was a Roman Catholic nun of the Franciscan order. Small of stature, but larger than life, she did not fit the stereotype of a nun. She spoke fluent French, English, and two dialects of Chinese. She was the principal of a school in Macao, and she was very much attuned to the secular world. The Franciscan order allowed Aunt Teresa a visit with her family every seven years. On her visits, she always took center stage. Among her nieces and nephews, four were physicians, but that did not deter her from always having something to teach us. One of the last times we saw her, she taught my brothers, cousins, and me to do acupuncture. On that visit, she introduced me to ear acupuncture and gave me a book titled *Practical Ear-Needling Therapy.* She also told me that a Dr. Wen in Hong Kong had great success using this form of acupuncture to treat drug addiction. There now is at least one similar clinic in New York, and its success rate exceeds that of methadone. Aunt Teresa further explained that there was a representation of the entire body on the ear, with specific points of the ear corresponding to specific organs. With this ear-needling technique, you could use an electrical detector on the ear, a detector that would sound off when it "read" a diseased organ, indicating which ear point to treat.

This was not the first time I had been intrigued by what acupuncture could do. In Taiwan, I had seen a patient who carried two symmetrical scars on either side of the lumbar spine. It appeared as if someone had branded him with two hot barbecue skewers.

He told me that ten years before, he had suffered from terrible back pain and was treated by a Japanese acupuncturist who not only needled his back but also held heat to the needles, causing the burns. Since then, his back pain had disappeared. This treatment was certainly economical compared to a lumbar laminectomy, I thought. As for complications, the only one I could think of was a potential infection from the burns. That risk pales, however, compared to the potential complications of a lumbar laminectomy: bleeding, infection, paralysis, and even death. In 1961, newspapers reported that the movie actor Jeff Chandler, while undergoing a lumbar laminectomy, had died from accidental injury to the aorta, the main blood vessel of the body. These thoughts had remained hibernating in my mind.

I had practiced emergency medicine for six years and seen my share of bad outcomes with drugs. There was the patient who took a muscle relaxant for a sprain and ended up with an allergic reaction, an exfoliative dermatitis that resulted in the skin peeling off her entire body. There was a colleague who had a simple tendonitis from weekend gardening; he took a nonsteroidal anti-inflammatory drug (NSAID) and ended up with kidney failure requiring months of dialysis. There were the cases of upper gastrointestinal (GI) bleeding among NSAID users requiring hospitalizations, gastroscopies, and even transfusions. There was a patient who came in with an intestinal perforation, an uncommon but dangerous complication of NSAID use. I was ready to explore alternatives.

Before Aunt Teresa's 1980 visit, I had dabbled in acupuncture but was not impressed that it was particularly effective. I had not realized that results come only after multiple treatments. Aunt Teresa's enthusiasm and instruction rekindled my interest. I began using a combination of ear acupuncture diagnosis and body acupuncture treatment on my co-workers in the ER, often with gratifying results. For the treatments, I used a small electric stimulator, given to me by Aunt Teresa, to which acupuncture needles could be hooked up with wires. One of my first subjects was a rather high-strung physician with shoulder pain. I needled him with the machine on low. He complained the current was much too strong. I reassured him, increased the current, and he calmed down. My next subject was a ward clerk who had chronic back pain. I administered the treatment in the same way as with the doctor. I had barely turned the machine on when my patient nearly leaped off the stretcher. I decided not to use electricity on him. Then I treated one of our nurses for neck pain, and she figured out the problem. "Pat, I think the dials on the machine are reversed, so high reads low and low reads high," she said. That should not have been surprising, I thought. The Chinese convention is to address people by their surname followed by their given name. Chinese words are written vertically and read from right to left.

I then began attending more acupuncture seminars. At one of these seminars, I heard that a school called the American College of Traditional Chinese Medicine would be opening in San Francisco in 1981. The school was going to teach Chinese herbal medicine as well as acupuncture. This was the opportunity I had been waiting for since 1962. I enrolled immediately. One of my physician colleagues in the ER asked if I was the only ethnic Chinese physician in the class. Indeed I was. He teasingly said, "That figures. Other ethnic Chinese physicians have better sense." With a chuckle, I replied, "Yes, I am well on my way to becoming a quack." But deep down, I believed this endeavor held a lot of promise.

Chapter 2

Elementary Traditional Chinese Medicine: The Organs

At the American College of Traditional Chinese Medicine (ACTCM), there were approximately thirty students with diverse career backgrounds. In medically related fields were a pharmacist and a registered nurse. Among the rest, career experiences ranged from secretarial to computer programming. I was the only physician. Our faculty members numbered six. One of the six, Dr. Yat Ki Lai, eventually became my lifelong teacher and mentor. Classes were held in the evenings and weekends. Our initial makeshift classroom was in a faculty member's house, where folding chairs were set up in the dining room. All the students had day jobs, so we usually came to class tired. Although classes began in winter, we kept the windows open to stay awake.

My early days at ACTCM were filled with disappointment and frustration. The philosopher John Locke wrote that a child's mind is like a blank slate on which you can write anything. For my class-mates with less formal medical training, the dogma of TCM was easy to accept. My slate was far from blank. Medical school and residency training had left their indelible imprint. I was not ready to accept ideas contradictory to what had already been deeply etched in my mind. What I heard in the lectures verged on heresy. As the other students nodded in acceptance, I was thinking, "This is all wrong." I was appalled, for example, when one of our first lecturers said that sinusitis could be treated with herbs and acupuncture. Sinusitis is an infection caused by bacteria. The only known remedies are antibiotics and decongestants for stuffiness. How could herbs and acupuncture replace them? Quite a bit later, I learned that some herbs have antibacterial actions, and acupuncture is very effective in decongesting the nose and sinuses.

Lessons began with TCM organs. They are classified as follows: the five solid (zhang 臟) organs are the heart, lung, liver, kidney, and spleen; the six hollow (fu 腑) organs are small intestine, large intestine, stomach, gallbladder, bladder, and triple burner (三 焦), which is not actually an organ but three body zones consisting of the Upper, Middle, and Lower Burners. A Westerner might think of these zones as different areas of the body where calories are burned. The Upper Burner consists of everything above the diaphragm, most importantly the brain, heart, and lungs; the Middle Burner consists of the organs in the upper abdomen, namely the liver, spleen, and stomach; and the Lower Burner consists of the colon, urogenital system, and lower extremities.

The hollow organs are regarded as mere conduits for expelling bodily waste. Most bodily functions are attributed to the solid organs, and teachings about solid organs were what caused me such consternation. The lectures were delivered in Cantonese Chinese followed by English translation. Since I understood both languages, the contradictions could not have been attributed to faulty translation. The descriptions of the heart and lungs were not too different from Western ones; however, for the other three organs—liver, kidney, and spleen—they were unrecognizable.

Heart 心

The lecturer began by describing the heart as follows:

> *"The heart is the essence, the overlord of all internal organs of the six fu and five zhang. It is the abode of the spirit, and must be strong against outside evil or disease. If the outside evil influence has penetrated the heart, the heart will suffer such damage that the spirit will leave, and the human organism will die."*

Although calling the heart the *overlord* sounded strange, I figured that *the abode of the spirit* was not so different from the Western idea that the heart was "the seat of the soul." In antiquity, both cultures thought the function of the mind resided in the heart.

> *"The heart's Qi [function] must descend, not rise. If the heart Qi rises, there will be heart pathology, as in the feeling of one's heart in one's throat. The heart governs the blood vessels and circulation and is manifested on the face and tongue. An insufficiency of heart Qi causes pallor, glassy appearance, anorexia, poor and congested circulation with a black color in the face."*

The description of heart Qi insufficiency could easily be that of a moribund patient with advanced heart disease.

> *"An increase in heart fire results in redness of the tip of the tongue, painful mouth, or sores of the mouth, restlessness, and insomnia."*

The association of the TCM heart with fire and mouth sores was a bit strange until we were introduced in our curriculum to the Five Phases system of TCM (see chapter 4).

Lung 肺

Next came the description of the lung.

> *"The lung governs Qi. The lung is the sea of Qi. It gets
> Qi from the outside atmosphere and from inside the
> body when food is transported via the spleen to the
> lung. The lung is subordinate to the heart. The heart
> mobilizes the blood but it depends on healthy lung Qi.
> The nature of lung Qi is descending. If lung Qi rises,
> there is dyspnea, cough, congestion, edema, and dif-
> ficult urination. It opens channels for water. It assists
> water to descend into the bladder."*

Lung Qi (literally, air that is inhaled) made sense to me as a Western practitioner. At this point, I could not grasp how the lung received Qi from food, but I found the rest acceptable. The description of what happens when lung Qi rises fits that of congestive heart failure, often accompanied by dyspnea, congestion, and fluid retention.

> *"The lung governs skin and body hair, which depend
> on lung Qi for moisture and nourishment. If lung Qi
> is weak, the skin and hair become dry."*

It is logical that poor lung function would impair oxygenation of blood, and therefore the skin and hair, suffering this loss, would become dry. We know that smoking is associated with premature aging of skin. I later learned that one TCM principle for treatment of skin diseases is to treat the lung.

Although I found some ideas a bit quirky, I still approached TCM teaching with an expectant attitude.

Liver 肝

When the lecturer began describing the liver, things began to change. The description bore no resemblance whatsoever to the organ that I knew as the liver.

"The liver is the general of organs; it strategizes, needs to flow, and dislikes obstruction," he said.

I could accept calling the liver a *general* and saying it *strategizes*, because the liver is actually an organ of metabolism, clearing the body of a multitude of compounds. What was this about *needs to flow*? Had the general now turned into a river? Where is the river going? This is ridiculous, I thought, but since I had already paid for my tuition and had come with the attitude that this system of medicine worked, I was determined to hear the teachers out before drawing any firm conclusions.

> *"If liver Qi* [function] *is congested, a person will anger easily, have chest and flank swelling and pain, and women will have irregular periods. If liver Yang* [force] *is rising upward, one will have headache and dizziness. If more severe, the eyes will ache, get red, and if even more severe, a stroke could ensue. Liver is closely linked with emotions. If liver Qi is deficient, the patient is easily frightened or angry. In America, there is a lot of liver Qi illness.*
>
> *It stores blood. If it loses this function, the patient will have insomnia, be easily awakened, and have fitful sleep or many dreams.*
>
> *It governs the ligaments of the body, flourishing in the finger and toenails, and exits through the eyes. If liver Qi is congested, it invades the Spleen. Symptoms are anorexia, diarrhea, and poor digestion."*

He was certainly not describing the liver as I knew it. But as I listened, it began to dawn on me that what he was describing was the sympathetic nervous system! We have a two-part autonomic nervous system that regulates involuntary responses. The parasympathetic part turns on for our vegetative functions such as digesting food. The sympathetic part is activated for fight or flight. This occurs when we face an urgent, stressful situation such as being chased by a wild animal, or in a modern-day setting, a potential head-on car collision. In these situations, the pupils dilate to enhance vision, the heart beats faster and stronger, blood pressure is elevated, and there is increased circulation to the brain. At the same time, circulation is diverted from the digestive tract to muscles, enhancing the ability to run or fight. In addition, sweating is stimulated to help cool off the body from the heat generated by increased circulation and muscle activity.

Some anatomy texts describe the adrenal gland as one big sympathetic ganglion (nerve cell) secreting epinephrine and norepinephrine (also called adrenaline and noradrenaline) into the blood stream. The resultant effect is similar to sympathetic nerve cells stimulating each organ. The TCM Liver then must include the adrenal gland.

The patient will have insomnia, be easily awakened, and have fitful sleep or a lot of dreams. Sleep disturbance occurs when there is heightened sympathetic activity.

If liver Qi is deficient, the patient is easily frightened or angry. The emotional link also fits the fight or flight mechanism. *A lot of liver Qi illness occurs in America* certainly fit. Just look at the American phenomenon of road rage.

Headache, dizziness, and possible stroke can all result from high blood pressure when there is excessive sympathetic or adrenergic activity.

Even the fact that the Liver *governs the ligaments of the body* made sense, as there is increased blood flow to muscles when the sympathetic or adrenergic system is turned on.

Interpreting the Liver in this way, I could understand the TCM syndrome called Liver Fire Uprising 肝火上升. The syndrome describes a patient who has low energy but is irritable. He may have a rapid pulse, sweat easily, and be light-headed. The description fit how I felt after having been up all night on emergency duty. The next day, my body was in sympathetic overdrive to compensate for the lack of rest.

Liver Fire Uprising (also called Deficiency Fire 虛火) is a very common condition. Women, during their reproductive years, lose blood with the menstrual cycle. Blood or fluid loss, when not replenished, tends to stimulate a sympathetic response. Symptoms of palpitation, insomnia, and irritability can further be augmented by the other stresses of modern life. Young women with such symptoms are often labeled neurotic or anxious. Chinese calming Liver Fire 疏肝 herbs such as Cortex Lycii Radicis 地骨皮 and Radix Stellariae Dichotomae 銀柴胡, which reduce the sympathetic response, in combination with other herbs such as Angelica Sinensis 當歸, which restore blood, can be good alternatives to psychotropic drugs used for these conditions. These same calming Liver Fire herbs are also useful for menopausal women with hot flashes, palpitations, and sleep disturbance.

I was stymied by the description of the Liver's *exiting through the eyes* until I connected the Liver with the sympathetic nervous system. When the sympathetic nervous system is stimulated, the pupils dilate. Pupillary dilation aggravates conditions like glaucoma. Western doctors often treat glaucoma with beta-blockers, drugs that block the beta-receptors of the sympathetic nervous system. In TCM, herbs classified as having the action of calming Liver Fire are used for eye diseases. Although they are not beta-blockers, these calming Liver Fire herbs work on the eye by decreasing sympathetic activity. Chrysanthemum 菊花, a calming Liver Fire herb, is often prescribed by TCM practitioners for painful, dry eyes as well as for hypertension.

When a TCM practitioner tells a patient that his illness is caused by a Liver problem, the patient assumes the practitioner is referring to the actual organ. My insight into the connection between the sympathetic and adrenergic systems and the TCM Liver enabled me to dispel this misconception. Greta, an attorney who had just moved from the East Coast to San Francisco, had a glaucomatous eye condition. She told me that an acupuncturist in the past had needled Liver points to treat the condition. She thought that there was a connection between the liver and the eye, and that perhaps there was something wrong with her liver. I explained to her that treating the TCM Liver was actually directing treatment to the sympathetic nervous system, not the actual organ. If we understand the TCM Liver to be the sympathetic nervous system, the treatment principle makes sense. In fact, Greta was taking beta-blocking eye drops prescribed by her ophthalmologist. I encouraged her to continue her existing treatment and reassured her that liver disease did not cause her glaucoma.

Ralph, a stockbroker, sought acupuncture for migraine head-aches. His primary doctor incidentally found that Ralph had abnormal liver functions. Further testing did not reveal the cause. Somewhere, Ralph had read that Eastern medicine attributed migraine headaches to a Liver problem. He reasoned that perhaps his abnormal liver studies were related to his migraine headaches, and that acupuncturing points designated to treat Liver would straighten out both conditions. In actuality, migraine headaches involve instability in blood vessel size. The Eastern medical con-nection with Liver is a connection with the adrenergic and sympa-thetic nervous systems, which regulate blood vessels. I explained to Ralph that I could use TCM Liver points to treat his migraine headaches, but the treatment would have no effect on his liver function tests because the TCM Liver is not the same as the organ we know as the liver.

When I heard that the Liver *stores blood,* my reaction was, Wrong! Although the liver, with its massive double circulation, contains a huge reservoir of blood, it is the spleen, not the liver, that has the main function of storing blood. I then began thinking about the history of Chinese medicine. The descriptions I heard were over three thousand years old, from a culture where dissection of the human body was taboo. Whatever anatomy physicians learned was likely the result of butchering livestock and poultry. They had probably observed that the liver was a blood-filled organ. It was understandable that they attributed the function of storing blood to the liver.

At this point, I made the first of several discoveries vital to my entire understanding and use of TCM. I needed to pay attention not so much to the names but to the description of an entity to figure out what it represented. If we reflect on the history of medicine, attributing functions erroneously to the liver and other viscera is not uncommon. Middle Eastern cultures believed that emotions originated in the liver. In Iraq, it is common for lovers to say, "I love you with all my liver." In her book *The Spirit Catches You and You Fall Down*, about the cultural clash between Hmong refugees and the American health-care system, Anne Fadiman points out that the Hmongs consider a weak liver to be the cause of mental illness (1997, 205–206). Even in the West, don't we say, "My gut tells me ..." when referring to our intuition?

Kidney 腎

When the next TCM organ was introduced, I rather enjoyed the challenge of trying to figure out what the ancient Chinese were saying. Each description became a riddle for me: "Here's my description. What am I?" When we came to the Kidney, I found hidden in the flowery language a multitude of meanings, ultimately comprehensible to the Western mind.

> *"The kidney is the secretary of state. It has light, strength, power, and finesse, because it stores the essence of life, governs bone, which produces marrow, which goes to the brain and flourishes in the hair, and externalizes in the ear. When the essence in kidney is abundant, the limbs feel strong, agile, energetic, and one hears and sees well. The hair is the flower of the kidney.*

If kidney Qi is deficient, there is lower back ache, soft bones, weakness, fatigue, dizziness, and forgetfulness."

If good Kidney function makes an individual feel *strong, agile,* and *energetic,* the description of Kidney Qi deficiency, with *lower backache, soft bones, weakness, fatigue, dizziness, and forgetfulness,* fits the aging process just about perfectly. I used to wonder about the *flourishes in the hair* and *externalizes in the ear* until it occurred to me that with aging, or a decrease in Kidney *essence,* the hair thins and hearing is impaired. The term *essence* 精 is sometimes used to mean semen. Since aging is the result of a progressive decline in reproductive hormones, it is evident that the TCM Kidney must include the reproductive system.

In the context of Kidney function representing reproductive hormones, how can *produces marrow, which goes to the brain* be explained? It made sense when I analyzed *marrow* and *brain* individually. *Marrow,* here, represents both components of bone: cortex as well as marrow. Keep in mind that Deficient Kidney Qi (function) means the aging process. Sometimes with aging, the bone marrow's ability to produce blood cells can decline. Anemia in a geriatric patient is investigated by first looking for a source of blood loss; if no source is found, then a bone marrow biopsy is performed to determine if the anemia is from decline in production of red blood cells. The other common bone condition of aging is osteoporosis, which is thinning of the bony cortex. Osteoporosis occurs when there is a deficiency in either male or female reproductive hormones. The Kidney tonifying (enhancing) herb Drynaria Fortunei 骨碎補 (literally, marrow tonifying) is a component of many herb prescriptions for a multitude of geriatric conditions such as anemia and back pain.

Regarding *brain,* we know that with aging, there is a decline in brain function typified by forgetfulness and, in extreme cases, dementia. Incidentally, there is a known link between dementia and lack of the hormone estrogen. To understand the description *marrow which goes to the brain,* I again remembered that many TCM descriptions came from observation. The brain is totally encased in a bony protective covering, the skull. Using only observation, the ancients probably thought that the two, bone and brain, were somehow interrelated. When they saw relationships between entities, the Chinese commonly used verbal metaphors like "going" and "flowing" to connect them, metaphors that sound foreign to Western ears. In ancient writings, the brain was considered an extraordinary organ, not fitting into the five zhang and six fu. Much of actual brain function was attributed to the heart. Only later did TCM relate emotions, thought, and memory to the brain. Similarly, the uterus was considered an extraordinary organ for childbearing and menstruation, but the complex reproductive system was attributed to the Kidney (Wiseman 1996, 73).

Further discussion of Kidney went this way:

> *"The bladder is the Provincial Governor. It takes orders from the kidney. Liquid is stored in the bladder, which waits for orders from Kidney Qi before it can come out. In an older person Kidney Qi is poor, and there is difficult or frequent urination."*

Perfect, I thought, the metaphor makes sense! The lecturer described quite accurately what happens when an aging male has an enlarged prostate gland, which impedes his urination. TCM just attributes this condition to poor Kidney Qi. Whenever patients in midlife complain to TCM practitioners about thinning hair, decreased sexual ability, and difficulty with urination, the patients tell me: "He told me I have weak Kidney Qi." I smile to myself and think, that probably sounds a bit more acceptable than just saying, "You're getting old."

Spleen 脾

"The Spleen governs digestion, absorption, and trans-portation of nutrients and water. Every part of the body depends on Spleen. After birth the Spleen nurtures body Yin [fluid] *and Earth* [see chapter 4, Five Phases]; *it is by nature damp. However, it hates to be wet.*

Spleen Qi [function] *must be rising to be normal. Only if Qi is rising does nutrition derived from food go all over. If the Spleen Qi is deficient, it results in anorexia, edema, diarrhea, which means there is dampness congested in the body.*

The spleen governs blood. It makes blood and regulates the circulation and direction of blood flow. If there is malfunction, the symptom is deficient-type bleeding. The Spleen governs muscle. This governance goes all the way to the mouth and flourishes in the lips. If the Spleen is in good condition, the person is muscular and lips are red. If the Spleen is in poor condition, there is decreased muscle tone, and lips are withered and colorless."

At present, we know that energy needed for cell life requires both glucose and oxygen. We also know that they come from two different sources. Glucose comes from the food we eat, and oxygen comes from the air we breathe.

In ancient times, without the knowledge of oxygen or of heart and lung function, the Chinese attributed both glucose metabolism and oxygen transport to the Spleen. They knew food was needed for energy, and somehow energy was connected with breathing and the lungs. Therefore, they postulated a two-step process: the Spleen transformed the ingested food to *Qi* (energy) *and blood* and then the Spleen percolated both up to the heart and lungs. They called this the up-bearing function of the Spleen. It is noteworthy that in both TCM and Chinese martial arts, the Middle Burner Qi (function) is of prime importance because of this notion that everything vital happens in the Middle Burner where the Spleen resides. Interestingly, when studying Russian, I learned that the word for abdomen is the same as the word for life. My Russian instructor explained that in antiquity, Russians also believed that everything vital resided in the abdomen where food goes.

The TCM Stomach is closely related to the Spleen. It has the function of propelling food downward toward the colon for elimination. This is called the down-bearing function of the Stomach. Actually, this mechanism is peristalsis. The parasympathetic portion of the autonomic system controls peristalsis. In TCM, then, the Stomach represents the parasympathetic nervous system.

Our lecturer said that if the Spleen's up-bearing function were lost, the symptoms would be *anorexia, edema, and diarrhea.* Up to this point, the TCM Spleen seemed to represent the upper digestive tract and the portion of the pancreas that secretes digestive enzymes.

The next area discussed was the Spleen's tendency to be damp but that *it hates to be wet.* In further studies, I discovered that many Spleen tonifying (enhancing) herbs have a diuretic action, so in a sense, they reduce *wetness.*

When our lecturer proceeded to talk about how the Spleen *governs blood,* he lost me. He said that the Spleen generated and regulated blood, and if the Spleen lost its function, bleeding ensued. I was taught that it is the bone marrow's function to make blood. Platelets and clotting factors are what control bleeding. The spleen is a filter and reservoir for blood. Perhaps, as in the case of the liver, the ancients observed the spleen to be a blood-filled organ and therefore assumed that blood must have been made in that organ.

Although I could translate some of what TCM taught about the Spleen, I was unable to find a unifying parallel for this organ in Western medicine as I had done with the Liver and Kidney, but

I was willing to be patient and wait to be shown. Up to this point, my impression was that the Spleen represented the digestive system. It was also involved in water metabolism and the clotting mechanism.

The epiphanies I received regarding the TCM Liver and Kidney fueled my determination to learn more. Books about the history of Chinese medicine further helped explain the strange-sounding metaphors and personification of TCM organs. In ancient writings, the human body was depicted as a microcosm, more specifically, a small country. The organs named, while sounding like ones we know, actually represent physiological systems rather than organs. The functions assigned to them are analogous to those of governmental officials, bringing order to the body as to a geopolitical state. The reference to the heart as the overlord, the liver as general, and the kidney as secretary of state then becomes understandable.

Chapter 3
Qi 氣 and Blood 血

Qi and Blood in TCM are considered the essential elements of life. The study of TCM must begin with a clear understanding of these two concepts.

Qi 氣

After learning about the TCM organs, we began to study the anatomical locations of acupuncture points and were given practical instructions in needling. Before inflicting discomfort on others, we needled ourselves on accessible parts of the body such as the leg or foot. I found it took nerve to needle myself. With my anesthesiology background, I experimented with first numbing the skin with a local anesthetic but discovered that the sting of the local anesthetic was worse than the actual jab of the acupuncture needle.

One day our acupuncture instructor demonstrated how to insert the needle into the correct point to elicit the response called *de Qi* 得氣 (attaining Qi). He told us that the endpoint was reached when the patient felt a strange, aching, full sensation. A student volunteered to be the patient, and the instructor demonstrated by inserting the needle with a quick thrust through the skin into his leg. As he probed deeper with the needle, he continually watched the volunteer's facial expression and asked if he felt that strange sensation. As the instructor went deeper, the volunteer began nodding and said he felt a sensation like "when I hit my crazy bone at the elbow." Then the instructor withdrew the needle and quickly covered the area with his hand to "not let the Qi escape."

How quaint, I thought. All the instructor did was hit a peripheral nerve, causing the sensation. That is how I used to find nerves when I did nerve blocks as an anesthesiologist. The difference was that after I located the nerve in a similar manner, I injected a local anesthetic into it. Modern research has shown that acupuncture points have an increased electrical conductivity because the points are either on nerves or myoneural junctions (the location where nerves join with the muscles that they supply). So stimulating nerves or myoneural junctions by needling them is what the instructor called *de Qi*. This business of covering the hole where the acupuncture needle was pulled out, as if plugging up a leak in a tire, seemed silly. Did the instructor actually believe the Qi would escape, and that he could plug it up with his hand? My curiosity about the widely used TCM term *Qi* was aroused.

The literal meaning of Qi is "air." When Qi is used in its literal sense, we can consider the two anatomical locations where air is present: the lungs and the gastrointestinal tract. Shortness of breath, then, is shortness of Qi 氣短, abdominal bloating is being swollen with Qi 脹氣, and passing flatus is passing Qi 排氣.

Lowering Qi 下氣

"Lowering Qi" is a treatment term commonly used in TCM. If we keep in mind that the literal meaning of Qi is air, we can understand this term. Conditions that require the Qi to be lowered are those in which the Qi or air seems to be going the wrong way: shortness of breath, burping, and abdominal bloating.

The ancient Chinese observed that people were normally able to breathe effortlessly. The Qi, or air, seemed to go down from the nose and mouth into the lungs. But when someone becomes short of breath, he needs to work at getting the air down into the lungs. TCM practitioners used treatments to help the patient's Qi go down. One of my Chinese patients, who had shortness of breath with exertion when walking up hills, told me, "My upper Qi doesn't seem to meet my lower Qi." 上氣不接下氣. At the time, her description seemed peculiar, but it became understandable when I studied TCM. The Chinese envisioned the air breathed in through the nose and mouth as the upper Qi, which went down to meet the air in the lung, the air they called the lower Qi.

To treat breathing difficulties in which the normal flow of air seems impeded, such as with cough, asthma, or heart failure, Chinese practitioners use herbal remedies for lowering Qi. The remedies facilitate breathing by dilating constricted bronchial tubes and blood vessels and decreasing the sensitivity of the cough reflex. Herbal prescriptions for colds and coughs usually include one or more herbs for lowering Qi, such as Pericarpium Citri Reticulatae Viride 青皮 (green tangerine peel). Acupuncture points that work on the sympathetic system, which dilates bronchial tubes, are also used to lower Qi.

As for the gastrointestinal tract, we know that peristalsis, the synchronized motion of the gut, controlled by the parasympathetic nervous system, propels food, liquid, and air. When there is dysfunction of peristalsis, the patient experiences bloating and discomfort. Western medicine calls this problem gastrointestinal dysmotility and prescribes pro-kinetic drugs to regulate the nerves to the gut. These pro-kinetic drugs stimulate the nervous system to increase peristalsis. The Chinese ancients observed that, normally, Qi (air) should move in a downward direction during digestion. If there was a problem with gastrointestinal motility, it seemed to them that the Qi was moving up instead of down. To treat such a condition, herbs for lowering Qi, such as Cortex Magnoliae Officinalis 厚朴 and Pericarpium Citri Reticulatae 陳皮 (dried tangerine peel), which regulate peristalsis, are used.

The herbal remedies are comparable to the Western pro-kinetic drugs.

Aside from its literal meaning, Qi can have many other meanings, depending on what word is combined with it. In the Chinese language, modifiers determine the meaning of a word. As an adolescent, I went on a low carbohydrate diet to try to lose weight. When I became ill, my mother told me, "We Chinese say you need rice Qi 米氣 to stay healthy. Maybe the reason you became ill was that you overdid it with your diet by eliminating rice, and you don't have enough rice Qi." At that time, I paid little attention to my mother's words, putting them in the category of old wives' tales. As a TCM student trying to analyze the term Qi, my mother's words came back to me. What is meant by "rice Qi"?

Types of Qi

There are five major types of Qi in TCM: Zheng or Right Qi, Yuan or Original Qi, Organ Qi, Ying or Nutrition Qi, and Wei or Defensive Qi.

Zheng Qi 正氣

"Zheng Qi (Right or Normal Qi)," the lecturer said *"is the fountain-head of all force and energy of life."*

The Chinese character for Zheng, 正, is made up of a horizontal line above the character for stop 止. It means "stop when the limit has been reached." (Wieger 1965, 266) The word *Zheng* is used to mean "in the correct place." For instance, if a picture hanging on the wall is a bit tilted, the Chinese say it is "not Zheng." If you are wearing a hat that is off kilter, you need to "push it back to Zheng." When there are many roads to a destination, the main road is the "Zheng" road. *Zheng* connotes correctness and normalcy.

I looked for the Western medical equivalent of Zheng Qi and decided that it is the mechanism of the body that keeps functions normal. The best equivalent word for this is homeostasis, which describes how the body tends to keep itself in balance. The autonomic nervous system is one example. Another is the body's feedback mechanisms that keep hormonal secretions in check. One of these feedback mechanisms involves the pituitary and thyroid glands. The pituitary gland secretes TSH (thyroid stimulating hormone), which causes the thyroid gland to secrete its hormone. When the blood level of thyroid hormone is adequate, the pituitary gland senses this and shuts off TSH production until the thyroid hormone falls below a certain level. I believe that these kinds of bodily checks and balances are what the ancients had in mind when they talked about Zheng or Normal Qi. The common translation of Zheng Qi as "Righteous Qi" implies that there is a moral aspect to the term. "Right" or "Normal" are more accurate translations.

Yuan Qi 元氣

Yuan or Original Qi is commonly believed to be Qi that people are born with, thus implying genetic makeup. TCM teaches that the quantity of Yuan Qi a person has will determine how well he recovers from an illness. Although genetics is a strong factor, the other determinant of health is environment. How well a sick patient fares depends on a composite of both factors; therefore, using genetics alone to explain Yuan Qi is inadequate.

If our genetically endowed ability to fight disease could be likened to a tank of gas, the concept might be easier to understand. Just as some vehicles have larger tanks than others, some people are born with stronger genes or a greater supply of Yuan Qi than others. If such people adopt unhealthy habits, however, they will have used up their Yuan Qi faster, similar to the way putting many miles in your car depletes the gas tank faster. At some particular time in life, when these people contract an illness, how they fare will depend on how much Yuan Qi is still left. The best Western equivalent I found for Yuan Qi is baseline function—how well someone functioned before getting sick. It is easy to understand that if a patient who smoked for years developed a respiratory infection, he would have less Yuan Qi and be less able to overcome this infection than someone contracting the same illness who had comparable genetics but who had not abused his body by smoking.

Organ Qi 內臟氣

"Organ Qi," our lecturer told us, *"is what mobilizes each organ."* The simple Western definition is organ function. It has been said that a human being is made up of one long tube that propels food from one end, the mouth, to the other end, the anus. As discussed earlier, the gastrointestinal tract, a very long tube whose walls are made up of smooth muscle, functions by peristalsis, where the smooth muscles contract and relax synchronously. Hormones and the parasympathetic part of the autonomic nervous system control this synchronous movement. These controlling forces are the Qi that "mobilizes" each organ. To treat constipation in the elderly, an effective herbal prescription consists of not only lubricating herbs but also lowering-Qi herbs such as Cortex Magnoliae Officinalis 厚朴 that stimulate peristalsis.

We are also made up of many smaller tubes, transporting secretions from one point in the body to another. Westerners call these tubes ducts. For example, the salivary ducts carry saliva from the glands to the inner lining of the mouth; oil ducts carry oil from the gland to the skin. What determines how much secretion is brought to an organ is the size of the ducts. The walls of these ducts are made of smooth muscle that can contract or relax to make the ducts smaller or larger. Just as with the smooth muscles in the gastrointestinal tract, the smooth muscles of various ducts are controlled by the autonomic nervous system and hormones. With hot weather, the sympathetic nervous system stimulates the sweat glands to produce more sweat. To accommodate bringing more sweat to the skin surface for cooling the body, the sympathetic system also dilates the sweat ducts. When we eat, hormones are secreted to stimulate salivation, and the parasympathetic nerves stimulate the saliva ducts to widen. All these mechanisms are included in the concept of Organ Qi.

When flow is obstructed, it is often because the secretions have become too thick to pass through the ducts. Such is the case with a salivary duct stone. Sometimes, if a person becomes dehydrated, the saliva becomes thick to the point that it forms a solid stone, blocking further salivary flow. This can occur in the elderly, whose mucous secretions may be diminished because of age, and this dryness is further exacerbated by medications causing dry mouth.

A patient in her fifties once told me that she had pain in her cheek area where the saliva gland is located ever since her recent gallbladder surgery. With my background in anesthesiology, I figured that her salivary duct most likely became obstructed from dehydration caused by several factors around the time of surgery. To facilitate intubation of the trachea (inserting a tube in the trachea that is connected to anesthetic gases), anesthesia patients are usually premedicated with drying agents. Post-operatively, they may receive medications to control pain and nausea, which may further dry them. I advised my patient to increase liquids and apply heat to the area, and the pain resolved. When the Chinese talk about Organ Qi flowing, I believe this system of transporting fluid in ducts is what they mean.

A Chinese aphorism describes movement through these ducts: "Blocked results in pain 不通就痛; unblocked results in no pain 通就不痛." This truism can be applied to conditions as varied as angina and the pain of kidney stones.

Ying Qi 營養氣

> *"Ying or Nutrition Qi is derived from food and drink, springs from the Spleen and Stomach coming from the Central Burner. Its main function is to generate blood and nourishment."*

This clearly must be food metabolism. Perhaps this is what my mother meant by "rice Qi." TCM views the Spleen as the main organ of digestion and absorption, the Stomach as the conduit for the passage of food, and the Central Burner as the location where all these functions reside. With new research findings, Western medicine is discovering that this system is far more complex than what we once thought.

Wei Qi 衛氣

About Wei or Defensive Qi, the lecturer said, *"It springs from the Stomach and Spleen, goes through the Upper Burner, travels between the muscle and skin, and also enters all organ cavities. It defends against outside evil."*

Wei Qi undoubtedly is the body's immune system. The components of the immune system can be divided into two categories: white blood cells and proteins (called immunoglobulins). The Chinese attributed the source of Wei Qi to the Stomach and Spleen. These two TCM organs are responsible for digestion. Normal digestion of food is needed to make proteins for immunoglobulins.

Another component of the immune system, white blood cells, are made in several different sites: the bone marrow, the lymph nodes, and the thymus gland. I believe the TCM concept of Spleen, rather than representing one organ, actually includes these various sources of the white blood cell components of the immune system.

Our complex immune system can be likened to a military operation. Both immunoglobulins and white blood cells fit into a strategic system of defending the body against outside invaders. Rather like border patrols, white blood cells and immunoglobulins are stationed at the body's points of entry: the skin and the mucous membranes of the mouth, anus, and genitourinary tract. Others travel in the blood stream like reconnaissance troops, looking for the presence of invaders that might have already entered the body. When a foreign invasion is detected, white blood cells send messages to the brain, which in turn directs the bone marrow, lymph nodes, and thymus gland to increase production of fighting white blood cells. The blood then carries the fighter white blood cells to the body site being invaded. Meanwhile, an arms race is occurring: the white blood cells made in the bone marrow are designing immunoglobulins, which can specifically identify invaders, capture and destroy them, and avoid collateral damage. Transport for all these components is by way of the circulation. But remember that at the inception of TCM teachings, the circulatory system was not known. The ancients thought that Wei Qi traveled between the muscle and skin. How this concept originated is discussed in chapter 4.

Meaning of Qi

After listening to all the varied descriptions of Qi, I began trying to explore its overarching meaning. The popular Western notion of Qi is that it is a mystical, elusive entity having to do with a life force or energy, understood only by the Chinese and incomprehensible to the Westerner. Since I am a native Chinese speaker familiar with all the varied usages of Qi in common parlance, I was unwilling to buy into this Western notion. My overriding impression while studying TCM was that at the time the system was formulated, the ancients knew less, not more, than we do now.

I again tried to imagine what it was like back when these TCM ideas were formed. Little was known about human anatomy or physiology. It was 2,500 years before Andreas Vesalius accurately described human anatomy and William Harvey described the circulatory system. The ancients knew of neither the nervous system nor the circulatory system. As the Greeks did with their mythology, the Chinese devised ways to explain phenomena. Whereas the Greeks used their mythical gods, the Chinese, living in an agrarian society, used what they saw in nature.

The Chinese character for Qi is made up of a rice (米) and a vapor (气) radical. For the Chinese, rice is a staple, essential for life, comparable to bread in the West. Vapor exists but cannot be sensed. Let us recall that the literal meaning of Qi is air. We cannot see, smell, hear, or feel the air we breathe, but we know it exists; and without it, we cannot function. My conclusion is that Qi is a general term that the Chinese used to explain phenomena they did not understand. An entity's Qi is simply that essential element it possesses that makes it function. Some may interpret it as "force" or "energy," which are plausible synonyms. I think that in the same way the Chinese arbitrarily assigned to organs such as the Liver, Spleen, and Kidney certain bodily functions, so too they assigned to Qi the cause of many phenomena, usually of a dynamic nature, whose mechanisms they didn't understand. A parallel might be the Greeks attributing thunder and lightning to the god Zeus, or the sky being held aloft by the god Atlas.

Qi as the Nervous System

Going back to the general principle in TCM that Qi must move in an unobstructed manner for proper health, I considered what physiologic phenomena involved motion. Motion occurs in the nervous system, via electrical impulses. In Western medicine, there are two nervous systems, the central nervous system and the autonomic nervous system. The central nervous system originates in the brain and extends down the spinal cord from which nerves emanate. The brain sends messages to the muscles by way of the nerves, like a telemessaging system. The central nervous system controls all voluntary movement such as walking and talking. The autonomic nervous system telemessages to our internal organs and blood vessels but can bypass the brain, making the system faster. A metaphor for computer users might be that the autonomic nervous system is like broadband. This system controls automatic functions like heartbeat, breathing, and movement of the intestines.

Neither nervous system was known when TCM teachings were written. In fact, the ancient Chinese described the brain as the "sea of marrow," connected to the spinal cord. Their observation that both the brain and spinal cord are encased by bone undoubtedly led them to associate the nervous system with "marrow." The actual function of the nervous system with its intricate messaging circuitry was attributed to Qi.

Qi as the Cardiovascular System

In TCM terms, Qi and Blood are often used together. I used to think that Qi represented the oxygen carried in the blood. Yet I knew the name for oxygen was not just Qi but Yang Qi 養氣. As I probed further, it appeared that when Blood and Qi were used together, Qi represented the cardiovascular system.

The lecturer said, *"Blood is intimately related to Qi. Blood and Qi are always used together. Blood is Yin and Qi is Yang. Qi is the general of the blood. Blood is the mother of Qi. Qi holds the blood and moves it. Qi, however, needs nourishment of blood."*

In Western medicine, we know that it is the cardiovascular system, consisting of the heart and blood vessels that holds and moves the blood. Although early writings indicate that the ancients knew that blood flowed continuously in a circle (Lyons 1987, 127), they lacked a complete understanding of how the cardiovascular system functioned. I imagined the Chinese ancients observing blood spurting out when livestock were slaughtered or when soldiers were wounded in battle and thinking, "Something must be moving this blood, and something must be containing it in the normal state. It must be Qi."

Furthermore, the *nourishment of blood* required by Qi must be oxygen and nutrients carried by the blood. This description fits the coronary circulation like a glove. The heart, while functioning to hold and move blood for the entire body, depends on the coronary circulation for oxygen, glucose, and other vital nutrients to supply its own muscle. When a heart attack occurs, one of the coronary arteries feeding an area of the heart is obstructed. Deprived of the oxygen, glucose, and other nutrients normally fed to it, the muscle in that particular area of the heart dies. This scenario supports the TCM teaching that "*Qi* (the heart) *needs the nourishment* (oxygen, glucose and other nutrients) *of Blood.*" It is a tribute to the Chinese ancients' keen observation that they saw the interrelationship of the cardiovascular system that they called Qi and the blood that is carried within it.

The herb Fructus Citri Sarcodactylis 佛手, commonly called Buddha's Hand, whose flower has the appearance of a hand, has the effect of relaxing smooth muscle. The walls of both the intestinal tract and blood vessels are made of smooth muscles. The smooth-muscle-relaxing property of this herb serves to relieve intestinal spasm and dilate blood vessels. In Chinese herbology, it is classified as a lowering-Qi herb. Similar to the way Western medicine uses vasodilators to open blood vessels in order to lessen the work of a failing heart, this herb can be used when there is lung congestion from heart failure. My teacher, Dr. Lai, used to warn, "Be careful when you use this herb; too much of it can break the Qi, and the patient will get light-headed and faint." I used to puzzle over his warning. What was meant by "breaking the Qi" to cause fainting? I then discovered that if I substituted the word "circulation" for Qi, it made sense. A high dose of this herb can dilate blood vessels excessively and in turn lower the blood pressure. If the blood pressure becomes too low, there will be inadequate blood flow to the head, thus causing the patient to feel light-headed and faint.

There is a symptom complex in TCM called Qi deserting with the Blood 氣 隨 血 脫, resulting from major blood loss. Its features include "bright white complexion, a rapid pulse that is forceless, … lowered blood pressure, and cold sweating" (Wiseman 1996, 151). Any Western physician would recognize this description as hemorrhagic shock. TCM explains that both the Qi and the Blood have deserted the patient. It is quite evident that Qi here refers to the circulation.

Blood 血

The TCM concept of blood is the same as the Western one, except the ancient Chinese believed that it comes from ingested food and liquid that somehow gets transformed by the lung and "construction Qi" to turn it red in color. They believed that bleeding was caused by blood flowing in the wrong direction, and the Spleen managed or directed the blood to flow in the correct direction. TCM divided diseases of Blood into three categories: Bleeding 流血, Blood Deficiency 血虛, and Blood Stasis and Ecchymosis 血瘀.

Bleeding

The term for bleeding is the same in both TCM and Western medicine. Bleeding is considered by both East and West to be a serious condition requiring treatment. There are hemostatic 止血 herbs used to treat bleeding. In fact, TCM practitioners recognized that certain hemostatic herbs were more effective than others in treating certain kinds of bleeding (Bensky 1993, 355–381). For nosebleeds, Chinese practitioners used Rhizoma Imperatae Cylindricae 白茅根; for bloody sputum and bloody vomitus, Rhizoma Bletillae Striatae 白芨; for bloody stools, Flos Sophorae Japonicae Immaturus 槐花米; for bloody urine, Pollen Typhae 蒲黃; for uterine bleeding, Folium Artemisiae 艾葉; and for wounds, Radix Pseudoginseng 三七. In fact, Radix Pseudoginseng is included in a well-known trauma formula called Yunnan Bai Yao. Chinese soldiers used to carry a supply when going into combat.

Blood Deficiency

The term "Blood Deficiency" is similar to the Western term "anemia," but there is a distinction. Blood Deficiency means a decrease in the total blood volume, consisting of red blood cells and plasma (the liquid portion of the circulating blood), whereas anemia is a laboratory diagnosis made by measuring the concentration of red blood cells relative to the plasma. Conceivably, a patient could be Blood Deficient from the TCM perspective and yet not meet the laboratory criterion for anemia from the Western perspective. This is true of many women who lose blood every month. Their blood loss may not be of a magnitude that is measurable as anemia. Their blood vessels have adjusted to the smaller blood volume by constricting. Using TCM diagnosis, however, they are Blood Deficient. Many have cold hands and feet and are intolerant of cold weather. Because of these changes, TCM would further categorize them as being in a Cold state (see chapter 5). The West subcategorizes anemia into types and causes, and treats accordingly. The East is less specific, but its herbal pharmacopoeia includes several tonifying (building) blood herbs such as Rhizoma Polygonati 黃精, Radix Polygoni Multiflori Thunb 首烏, Angelica Sinensis 當歸, and Fructus Lycii Chinensis 枸杞子 (also known as goji berries).

Blood Stasis and Ecchymosis

Regarding the concept of Blood Stasis and Ecchymosis, Eastern and Western medical views differ. While Western practitioners view thrombosis (abnormal clotting in blood vessels, such as leg veins, coronary arteries, or cerebral arteries) as a serious condition, they do not regard ecchymosis (bruising) from trauma as a condition requiring much intervention. For the early stage of bruising, Western practitioners use icing to constrict blood vessels and thereby stem bleeding. Thereafter, they merely allow the body's normal circulation to gradually absorb the bruised blood from the tissues.

The Chinese, on the other hand, view ecchymosis (bruising) to be just as serious as thrombosis, requiring the treatment called mobilizing Qi and Blood. After blunt trauma, if the volume of blood leaked into the tissue is large, instead of ecchymosis, we call the accumulation of blood a hematoma. Sometimes Western practitioners will evacuate very large hematomas with syringe and needle. If hematomas are left alone, scarring can occur, transforming the hematomas into hard masses. In some cases, these scarred-over hematomas can be mistaken for malignant tumors. A case comes to mind of a woman patient who had hit her chest against a steering wheel in an automobile accident. Months had passed, and she had forgotten about the accident. A physician happened to examine her, found a firm mass in her breast and thought she might have breast cancer. It was not until the tests for breast cancer returned negative that she remembered the accidental trauma to her breast. The ancients may have observed how bruises could change into hard masses, a rather alarming phenomenon, and concluded that ecchymosis required intervention. They felt that pooled blood anywhere blocked normal circulation. They believed that tumors were from internal blood stasis or ecchymosis. They also believed, but erroneously, that heavy menstrual bleeding with clots was caused by internal blood stasis, and the clots obstructed normal menstrual flow. In addition to bruising, sprains and strains also fall under the category of ecchymosis. The treatment principle of mobilizing Qi and blood arose from this belief system that all Blood stasis conditions required aggressive treatment, a principle that is distinctly Chinese.

Mobilizing Qi and Blood 行氣活血 to treat Blood Stasis 血瘀

Two key herbal components are involved in mobilizing Qi and Blood formulas. One component, moves Qi 行氣. Herbs in this category include Radix Ligustici Wallichi 川芎, Rhizoma Corydalis 延胡索, and Radix Salviae Miltorrhizae 丹 參. If we interpret Qi to mean circulation, their mode of moving Qi becomes apparent. These herbs improve circulation by dilating blood vessels. Improved blood flow accelerates the normal process of absorbing blood from tissues. The other component consists of herbs for dispersing Blood 散血, such as Semen Persicae 桃仁, Achyranthis Bidentatae 牛 膝, and Flos Catharmi 紅 花. Radix Pseudoginseng 三七 also falls into this category. Its medicinal action seems to be bimodal. In higher doses, it is used topically to stem bleeding, but in lower doses, it is widely used to disperse blood. These herbs hasten healing by breaking up clotted blood, facilitating its absorption. They may work on platelets or on breaking up fibrin, and are worthy of further study. The closest Western counterpart of these herbs is antiplatelet drugs. We can regard them as being beneficial in treating thromboses.

To treat traumatic ecchymoses, the Chinese routinely use mobilizing Qi and Blood herbal formulas in the form of liniments 鐵打酒. Many also contain Myrrha 沒藥, recorded in the Bible as one of the precious gifts from the three Magi to the Christ child. Most Chinese families keep a bottle of herbal liniment at home as part of their first aid supply. Various liniments are commercially available, usually named after the practitioners who concocted them with their special secret combinations of herbs. Some Chinese Americans say that the American Indians actually have the best liniments, made up of Native American herbs. I became a believer in liniment use when I once caught my finger on the hinge of a folding table while closing it. My finger instantly became black and blue and began to swell. I quickly applied some liniment to my finger in the form of a poultice, and in a matter of half an hour, the swelling and discoloration disappeared.

It became clear that my interpretation of Qi differed from that of mainstream Western thinking. I wondered if I could find a kindred spirit, someone whose thoughts about Qi concurred with mine. I sought out my friend and colleague Adeline Yen Mah, a retired physician who devotes her time to writing. She grew up in Shanghai and understood Chinese culture. She was just finishing *Watching the Tree*, her book on Chinese philosophy, which had a chapter on Qi. I asked her for a copy of that chapter, in which she writes, "Matter and energy are part of a single continuum known as the 'the quantum field.' The ancient Chinese concept of Qi then may be the modern equivalent of this quantum field, which is constantly creating and disintegrating matter at the same time" (2000, 103).

It was not in this complex explanation that I found affirmation of my own explanation of Qi but in the anecdote that followed. Mah wrote that when she was a child in Shanghai, her grandfather listened to news on a shortwave radio every evening at about seven. The news was broadcast live from the BBC in London, where it was twelve o'clock noon. Mah asked her grandfather how far away London was. He told her it was thousands of miles away, halfway around the world. When she asked, "How can their voices travel so far, so fast?" his answer was, "This is due to the magical Qi of the English. When you grow up, you must learn from them" (2000, 104). In the same way that the ancient Chinese attributed the functions of the yet undiscovered mysterious nervous system and circulatory system to Qi, Mah's grandfather attributed the mystery of radio waves to Qi. Qi, rather than being the elusive, enigmatic energy flowing through our body, as Westerners ardently believe, is simply a term used by generations of Chinese to refer to the mechanisms behind phenomena that they did not fully understand.

"No time for your health today will result in no health for your time tomorrow."

— IRISH PROVERB

Chapter 4
The Six Evils 六病邪 and
Five Phases 五行

My next big challenge at ACTCM was to unravel the mysteries of the Six Evils and the Five Phases. As with studying the TCM organs, I again needed to realize the historical background from which these concepts came and to appreciate how culture influenced Chinese thought.

The Six Evils

The Six Evils are Cold 寒, Fire 火, Summer Heat 暑熱, Dryness 燥, Wetness 濕, and Wind 風. During the Shang Dynasty (1800–1051 BC), the Chinese believed it was unhappy demons, the spirits of departed ancestors, that caused disease. Perhaps the living neglected to place food before their ancestors' altars, perhaps they failed to burn enough incense to honor them, or they had not offered enough otherworld spirit money for them to use. Getting sick was a kind of wake-up call from their ancestors.

Later, in the Chou dynasty (1050–256 BC), beliefs shifted. The ancients saw how climatic changes seemed to influence health and began to believe that evil spirits associated with changes in the weather were the cause of disease. At the time of these TCM writings, infectious disease was the scourge of civilization, but the actual agents of infection, such as bacteria and viruses, were yet to be discovered. The work of Louis Pasteur, Joseph Lister, and Robert Koch, defining the germ theory, occurred in the 1800s; the work of Alexander Fleming, Howard Florey, and Ernst Chai, ushering in the era of antibiotics, did not take place until the 1900s. With only the tool of observation, the ancient Chinese attributed causes to what they were familiar with: changes in climate, believed to be brought on by evil spirits; indiscretion with food or drink; and extreme emotions.

Cold 寒

According to TCM, Cold evil appears often in winter. It attacks people through the skin. Even today, although we know a virus causes the common cold, the Chinese often continue to attribute colds to not wearing enough warm clothes. Under the skin is where Wei or Defensive Qi runs. Our lecturer explained that the symptoms of external Cold are *"fear of cold* [chills] *and fever without perspiration."* To me, these symptoms sounded like the early stages of the flu.

Our ACTCM lecturer further explained that if the Cold evil overpowered the Defensive Qi, it could penetrate deeper, to the muscle layer, and then to the internal organs. With this progression, the patient would develop *"a high fever, thirst, and profuse sweating. The Cold evil then turned into Heat."* This description fit the progression from an earlier to a later stage of the flu, or, for that matter, of any infectious disease.

The idea that the Cold evil, most likely the flu virus, enters through the skin and penetrates into deeper layers sounded preposterous. It is well known that the virus enters through the respiratory tract. Yet, I could see how, intuitively, the ancients would have assumed that it penetrated through the skin. When you first come down with the flu, you feel chilly and have goose bumps on your skin. Then the muscles begin to ache before the sneezing and coughing begin. That the Defensive Qi, most certainly meaning the immune system, runs under the skin seemed equally absurd. If I followed the ancients' train of thought that the evil entered the body through the skin, though, it would be a logical corollary that the first line of bodily defense would also run under the skin.

TCM teaches that if the Cold evil gains entry into the internal organs, the evil is transformed into Heat, characterized by a high fever, thirst, and sweating. Most infectious diseases are accompanied by fever, so the meaning of internal Heat 內熱 is easy to comprehend. There was even a book (now out of print) called *The Heat Diseases,* written in English, which was all about the treatment of infectious diseases. The Chinese character, 炎, for the term "infection" or "inflammation" (no distinction was made between the two conditions because the cause of infection by microorganisms was not known), actually has two radicals for fire 火, one on top of the other.

I wondered why it was important to distinguish between the early "external" stage of the flu and the later "internal" stage. The reason, I found, is that the TCM treatment for each stage of an illness is different. In early stages of the flu, practitioners use acupuncture and herbs such as Ginger 生薑, Radix Ledebouriellae Sesloidis 防風, and Herba Schizonepetae 荊芥 to warm the body. In the later stages, when there is excess Heat, clearing Heat and cleansing Toxin 清熱解毒 herbs (also known as cold-cleansing herbs) like Folium Istadis 大青葉, Radix Isatis 板籃根, Fructus Forsythiae 連翹, and Flos Lonicerae 金銀花 are used. Most cold-cleansing herbs have either antiviral or antibacterial actions.

Fire 火

The symptoms of Fire were explained as *"thirst, high fever, profuse sweating, bloodshot eyes, reddened face accompanied by delirium, and a bleeding tendency."* With a severe infection such as meningococcal meningitis, high fever with delirium is common; so are hemorrhagic rashes. Fire, then, is the evil causing severe infectious disease. I noted that description and cause are often interchange-able in TCM.

Summer Heat 暑熱

Our lecturer listed the symptoms of Summer Heat as *"fever, profuse sweating, thirst, lethargy, dry mouth, cracked lips, constipation, and scant urine."* He went on to say, *"Summer heat evil can accom-pany wet evil* [inflammation accompanied by fluid overproduc-tion] *with an excess intake of cold drinks and raw food, resulting in anorexia, nausea, and vomiting."* The first set of symptoms of Summer Heat could fit either heat stroke or an infectious disease, but the second set, accompanying Wet evil, sounded more like an infectious gastroenteritis, commonly called food poisoning. What, I wondered, distinguished infectious gastroenteritis, an ordinary infection or Heat disease, to make it separately catego-rized as Summer Heat? It took a while for the answer to dawn on me. Whenever my patients travel to countries where sanitation might be questionable, I advise them to avoid eating cold raw food and encourage them to eat anything that is cooked and served hot. The reason, of course, is contamination. The heat of cooking will usually kill unfriendly organisms. I imagined what it must have been like 3,000 to 5,000 years ago without refrigera-tion. In the hot summer months, raw food left outside spoiled quickly and people became sick. So of course, the Summer Heat Evil must have been the culprit.

Dryness 燥

The list of conditions caused by Dryness includes *"a hacking cough; blood-tinged sputum; chest cavity pain; fever; dry nose, throat, and sinuses; and fever accompanied by dry mouth, dry skin, cracked lips, dry tongue, and extreme thirst."* All these symptoms typify any respiratory infection, from pneumonia to pulmonary tuberculosis.

Symptoms of internal Dryness include nausea, vomiting, diarrhea, diaphoresis, and bleeding. These symptoms describe an infectious disease such as gastroenteritis, which leads to dehydration. But dryness is a result, not a cause, of these conditions. Are cause and effect being confused? Then I remembered: the ancients were simply saying that the Dryness Evil caused the dehydration. An understanding of Chinese grammar helps explain seeming discrepancies in how Chinese terms are used. Nouns and adjectives are interchangeable in Chinese, so the same word is used for the adjective "dry" and the noun "dryness." Furthermore, with repeated usage, the term "Evil" was understood and dropped, and the descriptors Cold, Fire, Summer Heat, Dryness, Wetness, and Wind were used alone.

Wetness 濕

Understanding Wetness was a bit more challenging. Wet diseases involve abnormal fluid accumulation: the body either retains or produces too much fluid. Wet conditions in TCM include *"leg heaviness and edema, milky vaginal discharge in the female, cloudy urine in the male, dysentery, and eczema."*

Edema, or excess fluid retention, can have many causes, such as kidney failure, heart failure, or cirrhosis of the liver. Many times, Western medicine uses diuretics to treat it. In TCM, edema is considered Spleen Wetness. Some Spleen herbs such as Sclerotium Poria Cocos 荷苓 are diuretics. Simply stated, whenever patients had abnormal fluid retention, the ancients believed the Wet Evil caused it.

Fluid overproduction from inflammation is what vaginitis, cloudy urine, dysentery, and eczema have in common. In all these conditions, the body reacts, whether to an infectious agent or to an allergen, with an immune response. The immune response causes the pores of capillaries, which are the body's tiniest blood vessels, to open and leak fluid, resulting in tissue swelling and, sometimes, drainage. TCM classifies these conditions as Wet diseases. If the inflammation is from an infection, cold-cleansing herbs are used. If the inflammation is from an allergic reaction, such as with eczema, treatment is directed at controlling inflammation and the allergic response.

Wind 風

When it came to Wind, I was stumped. At ACTCM, I was definitely out of my element. Although I was used to being in the minority, being of Chinese ancestry while growing up in white America and being a female entering the male-dominated field of medicine in the 1960s, there had never been a time when I felt more isolated than when I was a Western-trained physician studying at a TCM school. I felt like Gulliver in the land of Lilliputians. No one spoke my language.

Perhaps only one faculty member could understand my question, "What is Wind in Western terms?" Dr. K. was a Western-trained surgeon from China. At the time of the Cultural Revolution when intellectuals and anyone suspected of harboring Western ideas were persecuted, Dr. K. was imprisoned. After ten years, he finally escaped and made his way to the United States. By then in his sixties, it was unrealistic for him to resume his past career, so he began to pursue work in TCM, a field new to him. Like me, he had to learn a completely new paradigm. Perhaps because of the years of imprisonment, he did not volunteer his thoughts too readily. When I asked Dr. K. what he thought Wind stood for, he told me that Wind described diseases that had a rather abrupt onset and tended to move around in the body.

In the West, diseases are classified according to etiology (cause) or anatomic (body) systems. Without knowledge of either, early TCM practitioners classified diseases according to what they observed. They must have noted how wind played havoc with nature. Hurricanes could lift off roofs and cause extensive destruction. Storms came suddenly, often without warning, and moved through an area rapidly and unpredictably.

An English translation of a classic TCM text, *Fundamentals of Chinese Medicine,* published years after my TCM training, describes Wind thus:

> Wind is the chief of a hundred diseases. It is light and buoyant by nature, and most easily invades the upper body and the fleshy exterior, causing headache, dizziness, red and swollen face and eyes. Wind often invades the lung, manifesting as nasal congestion, sore throat, and cough.
> (Wiseman 1996, 187)

The ancients observed that strong winds such as hurricanes seem to sweep things in an upward direction, lifting off roofs. They surmised that conditions affecting the upper part of the body were caused by Wind. Migraine headaches, sore throat, and respiratory infections are some upper body conditions attributed to Wind. A Chinese patient, while sitting in my office, described her symptoms that were typical of migraine headaches. As she talked, she remarked, "The headaches must be because of my being in the wind." At that instant, she quickly covered her head with her scarf as if that would protect her from a recurrence. Old beliefs die hard.

Just as the direction of wind is changeable, some diseases such as hives and arthritis seemed to migrate from one location of the body to another. Wind was also thought to cause them.

The sudden and destructive nature of strong winds like hurricanes or tornadoes led the ancients to think that Wind must be the cause of sudden and severe illnesses. Tetanus, a disease caused by a bacteria entering through a dirty wound, is called wound Wind 破傷風 in Chinese. The ancients observed that after such a wound, the patient would suddenly get violently ill. In the West, we hardly ever see this disease because we immunize against it.

Stroke, called Wind attack 中風, is also a condition with a sudden onset and of a severe nature, but the ancients observed that it seemed to come not from meteorological changes or external Wind but from some process within the body. So they explained these conditions as coming from internal Wind 內風. TCM practitioners must have seen the association between people with excessive Liver Yang and the tendency to get strokes. People with too much Liver Yang have an overactive sympathetic system, leading to high blood pressure. TCM explained that excess Liver Yang could be transformed to Liver Wind and lead to strokes. Westerners also recognize that high blood pressure predisposes people to strokes.

Wind, like Qi, is often used in combination with another word to expand its meaning: arthritis is Wind Wet 風濕; gout is painful Wind 痛風. Unlike Qi, which can connote desirable or undesirable phenomena, depending on its modifier, Wind usually connotes something pathological. Wind can overlap with other Evils as the cause of some diseases. For instance, either the Cold Evil or the Wind Evil can cause the common cold. Overlapping and even conflicting concepts, while unacceptable to the highly compartmentalized Western mind, is not a problem for the Chinese, who easily reconcile conflicting concepts.

After having overcome the hurdles to understand its terms, I questioned why TCM so tenaciously preserves all these antiquated notions about disease when many concepts have been supplanted by modern science. Why do practitioners still use the term "Liver" when it means the sympathetic system, or "Cold Evil" when they know it is actually the flu virus? I came up with two explanations. One is cultural and the other is pragmatic.

The Chinese are traditionalists. They tend to preserve the teachings from previous generations even when the teachings conflict with newer findings. This peculiarly Chinese custom can be attributed to the interrelationship of two cultural factors: the concept of Face and the practice of ancestor worship, both deeply engrained in the Chinese psyche. Face is the Chinese ideal of preserving a person's dignity. To save Face, you avoid humiliating or embarrassing a person. Face is what prevents a Chinese from telling you the truth when you ask, "How do you like my cooking?" Face is what prevents a Chinese from airing the family's dirty laundry in public. Face is what drives patients with unsatisfactory treatment outcomes to find another doctor rather than tell the first one his or her remedy did not work.

Ancestor worship came about from the ancient belief that the world consisted of two groups: the living, inhabiting the physical world, and the dead, inhabiting the spirit world. The two groups had an interdependent relationship. The dead depended on sustenance from the living in the form of food, burning incense, and spirit money. The fortunes of the living were determined by how happy the dead were kept. The Chinese buried their dead on high mountains so that the departed could be closer to heaven. If they could find a mountain whose shape was that of a chair, that was even better. It would ensure that the departed loved one was comfortable in his or her new abode. The living were obliged not only to supply the needs of their dead ancestors but also to preserve their Face. Therefore, anything taught by ancestors, even if refuted by newer discoveries, became immutable. The Chinese would rather be syncretistic and accept multiple, incongruous teachings than risk the chance of offending any dead ancestors.

The other reason why TCM keeps its ancient teachings intact is that its entire system of treatment is based on the ancient ways of diagnosis. Many treatments were developed empirically and worked. Even if the explanation for them was wrong, as long as they worked, and everyone was familiar with the terminology, why change?

There is, for instance, an entire class of herbs called quelling Wind 驅風 herbs. A common one is Radix Ledebouriellae Sesloidis 防風 whose Chinese name means "prevent Wind." These herbs are used for early stages of the common cold, hay fever, hives, and joint inflammation. They seem to divert blood flow away from the nasal passages to the skin and extremities. Interestingly, these same herbs are also classified as relieving-surface 解表 herbs because of the ancient concept that the Cold Evil gains entrance to the body through the skin surface.

In the West, we treat infections with various types of antibiotics, each type tailored to fight the bacteria that tend to invade a particular part of the body. We have a class of antibiotics for fighting respiratory tract infections and another class for fighting skin infections and still another for fighting infections in the intestinal tract or genitourinary tract. We classify these drugs by studying the bacteria that seem to gravitate to certain areas of the body. Similarly, the ancient Chinese had a compendium of herbs for clearing Heat 清熱. These herbs were further classified as to which types of bodily Heat conditions they were best suited. For respiratory infections, practitioners used Flos Lonicerae 金銀花, Fructus Forsythiae 連翹, and Folium Istadis 大青葉, whereas for intestinal and urinary infections, they used Radix Scutellariae 黃芩, Rhizoma Coptidis 黃連, and Cortex Phellodendri 黃柏. How were they able to determine these differences without a microscope or a lab? Their diagnostic tool was their sense of smell. Each type of bacteria causing infection gives off its own distinct odor. For the TCM practitioner, this ability to differentiate the type of Heat Evil by the whiff test became highly developed.

Five Phases 五行

While the Six Evils explain disease from the atmospheric perspective, the Five Phases or Five Elements Theory explains phenomena from an earthly perspective. This system, devised in 400 BC, attempts to explain all cosmic phenomena and their interrelationships. Its launching point is the recognition of five terrestrial elements: Wood, Fire, Earth, Metal, and Water. Each element has distinct attributes.

Wood 木 is the bending and the straightening …
Fire 火 is the flaming upward …
Earth 地 is the sowing and reaping …
Metal 金 is the working of change …
Water 水 is the moistening and descending to low
places …(Wiseman 1996, 7–8)

Diverse phenomena, such as season, weather, direction, animate development, color, flavor, organs, tissue, and emotions, are classified according to their similarity to the elemental attributes. Regarding organs, some classifications are more self-evident than others. The Heart, associated with blood, which warms the body, is assigned to Fire; the Spleen, involved with transformation of food to energy, is assigned to Earth, which transforms seed to fruit; the Kidney, understandably, is assigned to Water. Others are a bit more obtuse, such as the Liver being assigned to Wood and Lung to Metal.

The system does not stop with just classification. If it did, the older English translation of 五行 as "Five Elements" would be appropriate. Now it is felt that the more accurate translation of 五行 is "Five Phases," because the theory purports that there are interactions between the five elements, called the engendering 生, restraining 克, and overpowering 侮 cycles, rendering the system dynamic rather than static. Just as the elements interact, the TCM organs correspondingly interact with one another. The Chinese believed that disease begins with an imbalance in these interactions.

What is the relevance of this system to today's practice of medicine? While there are entire schools of TCM practice devoted to the Five Phases system, I have found it difficult to treat patients by strictly adhering to it. The Chinese mind is typically very supple. Like the bamboo when the wind blows, it will bend rather than break. When I was living in Taiwan, I visited an art studio, shopping for a present for my brother. One painting caught my eye,

Table 1. Phenomena Categorized According to Five Phases Theory

Phenomenon	Wood	Fire	Earth	Metal	Water
Climate	Wind	Heat	Dampness	Dryness	Cold
Color	Green	Red	Yellow	White	Black
Development	Germination	Growth	Transformation	Harvest	Storage
Direction	East	South	Center	West	North
Emotion	Anger	Joy	Pensiveness	Sorrow	Fear
Zhang Organs	Liver	Heart	Spleen	Lung	Kidney
Fu Organs	Gallbladder	Small Intestine	Stomach	Large Intestine	Bladder
Sensory Organs	Eyes	Tongue	Mouth	Nose	Ears
Tissue	Tendon	Vessels	Muscle	Integument	Bone
Season	Spring	Summer	Long Summer	Autumn	Winter
Taste	Sour	Bitter	Sweet	Pungent	Salty

but I had a couple of reservations. I told the artist, "Most Chinese paintings have a story behind them, and this one doesn't." He quickly proceeded to spin out a story for me about the man in the painting. I then said, "I like it except for the colors; they are a bit too dark." The artist obligingly whipped out his paintbrush and dabbed some white snow on the canvas. The painting is now gracing a wall in my brother's home. The left brain in a Chinese

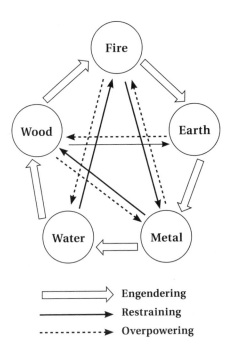

Fig. 1. Five Phases Interrelationships.

is permissive. It allows his right brain to bend anything to fit a metaphor. But even the staunchest devotee of the Five Phases system has to admit that adding an extra season just to fit them into the pattern of five is a bit contrived. Treating every patient's condition using this paradigm is likewise a strain. There is a limit to how far any metaphor can be carried.

Some schools of acupuncture have successfully applied the engendering and restraining cycle to selecting points for needling. The system categorizes herbs by their taste. While there is a relationship between an herb's taste and its therapeutic properties, finding a correlation between taste and the corresponding organ can also be a strain. Modern books on TCM also point out limitations of the system (O'Connor 1981, 18; Wiseman 1996, 13–14). Nevertheless, the Five Phases Theory so permeates Chinese thought and customs that I realized I needed to be familiar with it as I explored Chinese medicine.

Having studied the Six Evils and Five Phases, my journey into TCM had taken me to ever wider vistas. I was learning not only Chinese medicine but also Chinese history, culture, and philosophy. It was turning out to be a far richer experience than I had anticipated.

Chapter 5
The Eight Entities 八大綱

For several consecutive years in the 1980s, I served on my hospital's medical quality assurance committee. Our purpose was to analyze hospital cases with less than optimal outcomes and make recommendations for improving the quality of care. One year the committee observed that the hospital autopsy rate was consistently dropping. Ours was a teaching hospital involved in training residents. It was important to maintain a certain autopsy rate for teaching purposes. We brainstormed what factors were influencing families to grant or refuse autopsies. My charge was to research cultural and ethnic biases as factors.

To research the Chinese population, I interviewed my Chinese friends and patients on the subject. The message I kept hearing was that the Chinese prefer to be left whole. The Chinese have a revulsion to being cut, either in life or in death. One patient quoted her mother as saying, "I want to die with all my body parts intact." A Chinese surgical colleague told me that when he performed a limb amputation, he commonly saved the limb for the family to eventually bury with the patient. I was reminded of the elaborate burial sites discovered in Xian where the emperor was buried with life-sized statues of an entire army.

The Influence of Taoism 道教

Later, as I read more about the history of Chinese medicine, I discovered what a profound influence Taoism had on it. Taoism's basic tenet is that there is an order to the universe. That order is maintained by a balance of dualistic forces. Any disruption of that balance results in a catastrophe. The role of man is to live in harmony with that order, the Tao. If anything adverse happens to a person or his family, a Taoist believer assumes that somehow he must have done something by either commission or omission to disrupt the harmony of the Tao. An individual is considered a microcosm, therefore all Taoist principles apply to him as well in regard to health and disease. Being aware of this mindset has helped me to better understand my Chinese patients.

A Western physician colleague once commented that Chinese patients don't believe in chronicity of disease. They seem to loathe the idea of taking maintenance drugs such as antihypertensives and often stop the drugs once they are told their blood pressure has become normal. From a Taoist perspective, illness comes from an imbalance in dualistic forces; once the balance has been restored, normality should persist.

A family I knew dealt with a member's death from a heart attack by consulting with an oracle who told them the death occurred because they had painted their house the wrong color. No consideration was given to the patient's years of chain smoking. To a Westerner this may sound absurd, but not to a Taoist.

Taoism's pervasiveness runs deep. Many Chinese are not Taoists, but they are still influenced by its thinking. They seem to feel more culpable than other patients for abnormal test results. Chinese patients who test high for cholesterol often exclaim, "Why do I have high cholesterol? I hardly eat any fat." Less familiar with genetic predisposition to high cholesterol, they subconsciously think their adverse cholesterol report was caused by something they did. When my Chinese patients are diagnosed with a serious disease such as cancer, they often ask about what they should or shouldn't eat. To a Western-trained physician, the question seems irrelevant, but not to someone steeped in the Taoist worldview.

Taoism idealizes wholeness and forbids anatomical dissection. Consequently, the ancient Chinese were unfamiliar with human anatomy. Taoism, coupled with the Chinese custom of Victorian-like modesty, predestined TCM's approach to be noninvasive. Prudishness was carried to such a point in ancient times that women did not visit physicians, who were usually male. Instead, their husbands used a doctor's doll, a carved ivory representation of a nude woman lying on her side. The husband would describe his wife's symptoms to the doctor, pointing to the ailing part of the anatomy on the doll. Based on that information, the doctor would diagnose and treat the patient. This practice continued until China became a republic in the twentieth century when, under the influence of the American-educated Madame Chiang Kai-shek, the practice was banned.

In imperial times, a court physician was not even allowed to touch a female member of royalty. If a princess became ill, the physician was allowed to feel her pulse only indirectly. This was done via a string bound to her wrist and extended to another room where the physician sat to study the pulsations. This seemed so incredible to me that I sought verification from several sources. One of them was a TCM practitioner who came from a long line of TCM physicians and whose grandfather had been a court physician during the Qing dynasty. He told me that because diagnosing princesses was such an arduously difficult assignment, usually only the best among the court physicians was chosen to treat them.

Court physicians were considered dispensable and were readily beheaded if their diagnosis or treatment was not to the emperor's satisfaction. During the Han Dynasty in the second century AD, the emperor's physician was the famous Hua Tuo 華佗. He is considered the father of surgery in China. The emperor ordered him beheaded because he did not like the diagnosis of brain tumor Hua Tuo had given him. I often thought how foolish the emperors were to kill off their best doctors. They could not have been that easy to replace.

Understandably, Chinese physicians honed their skills very carefully. Like blind people, who develop a heightened sense of touch and hearing to compensate for their handicap, Chinese physicians, with the limitations imposed by cultural mores, learned to develop noninvasive methods of diagnosis and treatment to a far greater degree than Western physicians ever did. For them, the only tools available consisted of accounts of the patient's history coupled with keen observation, which included tongue diagnosis, pulse diagnosis, and the use of their four senses of sight, hearing, smell, and touch. It used to puzzle and annoy me that my Chinese patients insisted on bringing me a sample of their stool even when I told them it was not necessary. I now realize that my patients' practice was a holdover from the TCM custom of smelling excreta as part of the physical diagnosis of disease.

In the West, everything is compartmentalized, whereas in Chinese culture, all elements of life blend together. With the Taoist concept of wholeness, lines drawn between various disciplines are indistinct. Medicine merges with martial arts, religion, and diet. Interrelationships are perceived between the patient and his internal as well as external environment. Elements of a patient's internal environment include his constitution; his history—such as a severe illness, surgery, or trauma—which might cause weakening in certain organ systems; his food and alcoholic intake; and his spiritual and emotional state. For women, the timing of their menstrual cycles and whether they are pregnant are also considered part of the internal environment. The elements of a patient's external environment include the stresses of daily life and the season with its climatic changes. In today's setting, pollution must be considered as well.

My teacher and mentor, Dr. Lai, once saw a patient with kidney failure. When I asked him what the cause of the kidney failure was, he said that the patient was holding three jobs and worked himself to the ground. My reaction was, That doesn't answer my question. I needed to know what his renal biopsy showed, what was the basis of his disease on a cellular level. I realize now, from an Eastern medical perspective, the patient's overwork was a major factor.

A patient from northern China once showed Dr. Lai an herbal prescription he brought from his home province in order to get a second opinion. Dr. Lai is a native of Canton, a southern Chinese province with a temperate climate. He astutely noted that the prescription contained far more spicy-warm types of herbs than he customarily prescribed. He explained that in northern China, the weather is very harsh and cold. Northern Chinese herbalists habitually prescribe more warming herbs than southern Chinese herbalists do. He said that since the patient now lived in San Francisco, where the climate is temperate, the spicy-warm components of the prescription needed to be scaled down.

The Eight Entities: Four Pairs of Dualities

Yin/Yang

Out of Taoism evolved the concept of Yin and Yang. These two words represent the two contrasting sides of a prominence, such as a hill or mountain. Yin is the dark, cool, and moist shady side; Yang is the bright, warm, and dry sunny side.

The Chinese observed that throughout the cosmos there seemed to be a dualism requiring balance. In the field of physics, each atom has a positive and negative charge that balances

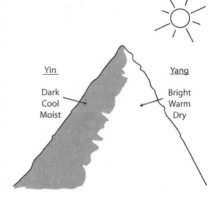

the other (an atomic explosion occurs when they are separated). In visual art, you need both light and shade for contrast. The sun heats; the wind cools. Winter is followed by spring. There is no such thing as a vehicle with an accelerator but no brake. This truth also applies to our bodies. We are female or male. We have a set of muscles that flex and another set that extends. We have a sympathetic and a parasympathetic nervous system. Our hormones have a turning-on and a shutting-off mechanism. Our blood stays in our blood vessels in a liquid form, but if we did not have a clotting mechanism when wounded, we would bleed to death. The Chinese have categorized all these dualistic forces as belonging to either Yin or Yang.

It is remarkable that the Chinese could condense all phenomena into this one simple concept. What comes to mind are the words of a sage Chinese physician who said, "It is simple but not easy." Whenever there was a disturbance in nature, the Chinese attributed it to an imbalance in Yin and Yang. Table 2 shows some dualities in medicine that fall into the Yin/Yang system of categorization.

Table 2. Yin/Yang Categorization of Common Conditions

YIN	YANG
Female	Male
Cold	Hot
Moist	Dry
Parasympathetic	Sympathetic
Depression	Mania
Hypometabolic	Hypermetabolic
Anti-inflammation	Inflammation
Anti-clotting	Clotting
Flexion	Extension
T Suppressor Cell	T Helper Cell

Recent medical literature reflects an increasing awareness among scientists of dualistic forces at work in the human body that need to be balanced for normalcy. In TCM, they would be considered Yin/Yang dualities.

The story of COX-2 inhibitors is a prime example. In our aging population, degenerative joint disease is commonplace. Western medicine relies heavily on nonsteroidal anti-inflammatory drugs (NSAIDs) to treat this chronic problem. While the drugs are effective in reducing the pain and inflammation of arthritic conditions, they are well known to carry the risk of stomach ulcers and GI bleeding. The reason for this adverse effect is that the older NSAIDs blocked the production of hormones called prostaglandins. Some prostaglandins cause inflammation, so blocking them was good for arthritis, but some prostaglandins protect the lining of the stomach, so blocking them was bad for the stomach. Traditional NSAIDs are known to block both enzyme pathways involved in prostaglandin production. These two pathways have been named COX-1 and COX-2 for short. Since prostaglandins mainly from the COX-2 pathway caused inflammation and prostaglandins from COX-1 protected the stomach, drug researchers thought that developing an NSAID that selectively blocked only the COX-2 pathway would be ideal. Such a drug would give the patient relief from the pain of inflammation without causing stomach ulcers or bleeding. Their efforts resulted in the development of COX-2 inhibitors.

Table 3. Yin/Yang Duality of the COX-1 & COX-2 Pathways

COX-1 Pathway	COX-2 Pathway
Protects stomach (Yin)	Causes inflammation (Yang)
Thromboxane—promotes blood vessel occlusion (Yang)	Prostacyclin—discourages blood vessel occlusion (Yin)

For a while, it seemed as if the COX-2 inhibitor was going to be the ideal NSAID. Western medicine further found a link between inflammation and colon cancer. It seemed people who used NSAIDs were less likely to develop colon cancer. Therefore, a study was begun to look for the protective effects of COX-2 inhibitors against colon cancer. A large number of patients, all prone to colon cancer, were randomly given either a COX-2 inhibitor or a placebo. The study was to test, after three years, if there was a difference between the two groups' development of colon cancer. Partway through the study, however, they discovered that people in the group receiving COX-2 inhibitors developed significantly more heart attacks and strokes than those in the placebo group, and the study was stopped. The COX-2 inhibitor drug, Vioxx (Rofecoxib), was voluntarily pulled from the market by its manufacturer (Bresalier, et al. 2005). A more recent study with another COX-2 inhibitor drug, Celebrex (Celecoxib), was completed and showed that subjects taking the drug did have a lower rate of colon tumors but had a higher rate of adverse cardiovascular events. Because of this risk, the drug is not recommended for prevention of colon cancer (Bertagnolli, et al. 2006).

A recent hypothesis was formulated to explain this adverse effect of COX-2 inhibitors. In nature, a prostaglandin called thromboxane, produced through the COX-1 pathway, causes platelets to become stickier, blood vessels to constrict, and the blood vessel wall muscle to grow—all factors that lead to blockage of blood vessels. These effects are normally balanced by prostaglandins called prostacyclins, made through the COX-2 pathway, which have the opposite effect. Prostacyclins discourage platelet stickiness, dilate blood vessels, and discourage the blood vessel muscle wall from growing. When the COX-2 pathway is blocked, prostacyclin production is blocked, and the effects of thromboxane then predominate, making patients more prone to heart attack and strokes (Solomon, et al. 2005). In Eastern terms, thromboxane made through the COX-1 pathway is Yang, and prostacyclin made through the COX-2 pathway is Yin. A balance of the two is needed to maintain normalcy in blood vessels.

In overwhelming infections, such as with meningococcal meningitis, sometimes the patient's own immune response is so exuberant that it actually harms the patient. It's as if the body goes overboard in its response to infection, and the excessive production of mediators of inflammation to fight the bacteria cause the host to become sicker. For these cases, Western practitioners use steroids to tone down the host's unchecked inflammatory response. Recently, medical researchers discovered that a Yin/Yang duality exists in the normal immune response. Some host immune cells make not only inflammatory cytokines but also anti-inflammatory cytokines to balance the response. In fatal cases, however, these bimodal adaptive immune cells that can dampen inflammation die in large numbers, leaving a heightened, unchecked inflammatory response (Hotchkiss and Karl 2003).

Another syndrome receiving much attention, especially with Iraq war veterans, is post-traumatic stress disorder (PTSD). A journal article describes the condition thus: Patients with PTSD have an inordinately prolonged reaction to a traumatic event. They have hyperarousal and frequently relive the event. Researchers found that sufferers of PTSD have abnormally low cortisol levels. In the presence of low cortisol levels, norepinephrine, a fight or flight hormone, acts on the nervous system unchecked. The effect of norepinephrine not balanced by cortisol leads to a constant panic-like state (Yehuda 2002). The TCM observer would interpret PTSD as an imbalance in Yin and Yang. The Yang of norepinephrine is excessive relative to the low Yin level of cortisol.

Besides Yin and Yang, the Chinese established three other pairs of dualities: External/Internal, Cold/Hot, and Solid/Deficient (also called Substantial/Insubstantial). The four pairs of dualities make up the Eight Entities. The Eastern way of disease classification is distinct from the Western way. The East purports that disease originates from an imbalance in the dualistic forces that operate to maintain normality. Eastern practitioners classify diseases in terms of which force is in excess or deficient causing the imbalance. The classification is descriptive in nature. TCM treatment is directed at reversing the imbalances by tonifying (replenishing) the deficiencies. If the patient has an excess of Yang, Yin-promoting treatment is used. If the patient has excess Heat, cooling treatments are used. The key to TCM diagnosis is to find the imbalances.

Yin 陰

In TCM, there are four kinds of body substance: Qi, Blood, Essence 精, and Fluid. Qi and Blood have been discussed in chapter 3. Essence 精 refers to sperm and ova, the sources of life. A common Chinese term, Jing Shen 精 神, meaning mental alertness, is a composite of the Chinese words for essence and spirit. Western and TCM practitioners alike recognize that mental alertness is manifested in the eyes. Fluid is everything in liquid form and belongs to the Yin category of the Yin/Yang paradigm.

When we eat, we salivate, and our digestive juices begin to flow. The entire lining of the ear, nose, throat and respiratory tract secretes a filmy liquid called mucous. These fluids have various antibodies protecting us from infections. All these normal fluids are Yin fluids. A deficient supply of Yin fluids causes disease. In a condition called Sjogren's syndrome, the glands secreting fluids throughout the body stop functioning. People with this condition have very dry mouths and are prone to tooth decay because they lack protective saliva.

One of my patients, Dan, was prone to getting prolonged bouts of coughing after having a cold or the flu. One season, he came to see me at the onset of his flu. I asked him when and how it started. He was able to pinpoint the exact time. It was after a very spicy Szechuan dinner. "As soon as I got home, I could feel my throat getting dry and hurting," he said. From the TCM perspective, Dan suffered from a loss of Yin fluid, caused by the spicy food, and as a result, he became ill. The TCM treatment he needed was to restore Yin fluid with herbs such as Folium Eriobotryae 枇杷葉 and Cortex Mori Radicis 桑白皮 as well as cold-cleansing herbs for his flu.

Yin fluid also represents the entire body's normal state of hydration. In most cases, Yin fluid connotes a good and normal fluid as opposed to Wet Evil, which connotes pathologic fluid.

Yang 陽

Yang is on the other end of the spectrum. If Yin represents the parasympathetic nervous system, Yang represents the sympathetic nervous system, which gears the body for fight or flight. It causes the body to be at full alert, with heightened senses, augmented heartbeat and breathing, and so on. With trauma, Yang forces stimulate clotting to go into high gear. In an immune response to outside invasion, Yang forces predominate. Such potent chemicals as interferon or tumor necrosis factor fall into the Yang category. Any inflammatory response also falls into the Yang category.

Heat/Cold

Heat 熱

The entities of Heat and Cold are similar to Yin and Yang, Heat being Yang and Cold being Yin.

Our lecturer described patients with Heat conditions as being *"restless, with red lips, red face, talkative, thirsty, constipated, having a rapid strong pulse, and often having fever."* All infectious diseases fall into this category. They are treated with cold-cleansing herbs, which have antibacterial, antiviral, antipyretic, and anti-inflammatory actions. In addition to infectious diseases, Heat conditions can include such disparate states as dehydration, hyperthyroidism, and mania. The latter conditions are treated with another type of "cold or cooling" herbs that act to decrease sympathetic action and stimulate parasympathetic action.

Cold 寒

Cold conditions, on the other hand, are those in which "*the patient is quiet, pale, with cold extremities, not thirsty, prefers warm liquids, likes to sleep curled up, and has an aversion to cold.*" The conditions I could think of that fall into this category are hypothyroidism, dysmenorrhea, and migraine headaches, all seemingly disparate conditions from a Western perspective. To treat Cold conditions, TCM practitioners use warming herbs, which tend to improve circulation.

It used to puzzle me when Chinese patients asked me if their cough was a Cold 寒咳 or Hot cough 熱咳. There is no such distinction in Western medicine. After studying TCM, it occurred to me that a Hot cough described an acute respiratory infection, whereas a Cold cough is one that lingers after the acute infection, characterized by fever and colored sputum, has ended. In retrospect, a lingering Cold cough was what I had after my pneumonia. Western medicine now calls it hyperactive airway disease. The scientific explanation for a Cold cough is that after an acute respiratory infection, the lining of the bronchial tubes becomes injured. The normal cilia (hairs), which help sweep away debris, and the mucous secreting glands, which help lubricate the bronchial passages, have not totally recovered their functions. For that reason, the cough reflex becomes hypersensitive, and coughing occurs when there is any increase in the air turbulence in the bronchial tubes caused by breathing cold air, talking, or laughing. The Western treatment principle is to dilate and relax the bronchial tubes with inhaled medications commonly used for asthma.

For a Hot cough, the TCM treatment principle is to clear heat 清熱, clean the toxin 解毒, rid the sputum 去痰, and stop cough-ing 止咳 by using "lowering lung Qi 下肺氣藥" herbs. For a Cold cough, the TCM prescription includes the aforementioned but omits the "clearing heat and cleaning toxin" herbs, and, in order to restore normal mucous secretions, adds herbs to "promote lung Yin 養肺陰."

To the Chinese mind, determining whether something is Hot or Cold is of prime importance, because it determines what type of treatment to choose. Moreover, since the Chinese medical paradigm includes food, patients want the information to guide them in food selection. If someone has a Hot type of illness, he should eat cool 涼 or cold type foods, and if he has a Cold type of illness, he should eat warming 溫 foods (see chapter 11).

Internal/External

After I learned about Cold Evil, the Western equivalent being the flu or other viruses, and the TCM explanation of their mode of entry into the body, the concept of Internal/External was easy to understand. The dual entities of Internal and External describe the early and late stages of an infectious disease.

Internal 內

The ancient Chinese believed that infectious agents, such as the flu virus, entered the body through the skin. If the Wei Qi (immune system) were not strong enough to defend the body against it, the virus would advance by invading deeper into the internal organs. Recently, a friend told me her mother had a bout of prolonged fever and consulted a TCM practitioner for it. Curious as to the cause, I asked what the TCM diagnosis was. The practitioner told my friend's mother she had Internal Heat. That answer failed to satisfy my Western mind, but I now realize that the explanation is as far as this ancient method can go.

External 外

Whereas Internal is a more advanced stage of an infectious disease, external refers to an early stage of an infectious disease. This classification is needed because TCM treatment is based on the disease stage. In the early, External stage, "surface relieving" herbs that improve circulation to the skin and extremities are used. In a more advanced stage, "clearing Heat and cleaning toxins" herbs are used.

Solid/Deficient

When these two entities were derived, it was in the context of infectious diseases.

Solid 實

A Solid condition describes what happens when someone has an acute infection and his body mounts an immune response to it with fever, rapid heart rate, and so forth. Blood Stasis and ecchymosis conditions (see chapter 3) are considered solid. Most tumors and cancers are similarly called Solid diseases.

Deficient 虛

A Deficient condition occurs when the body is weakened, fatigued, and enervated. In antiquity, this condition most commonly occurred as the aftermath of a serious infectious disease. Addison's disease, or adrenal gland insufficiency, with symptoms of severe weakness, fatigue, and lightheadedness, can be considered the extreme version of the Deficient state. Addison's disease can occur after a bout of tuberculosis where the infection destroys the adrenal gland. In addition to describing generalized debility, Deficiency can describe poor organ function. Someone with weak lungs, for example, is said to have lung Deficiency. The term is also used to describe an abnormally low level of a body substance, such as Yin Deficiency or Blood Deficiency.

After learning about the Eight Entities, I could not help wondering, since so much of TCM is about infectious disease, how is it relevant today, when we can treat infections so easily? If I had a patient with a urinary tract infection or strep throat, I would simply prescribe antibiotics, and the patient would begin to get better within forty-eight hours. Why revert to prescribing herbs? Herbs had to be boiled like a soup. Besides, most of these concoctions tasted so terrible. It seemed so impractical. My next task was to find out how TCM applied to contemporary life.

"The superior doctor prevents sickness; the mediocre doctor attends to impending sickness; the inferior doctor treats actual sickness"

— CHINESE PROVERB

Chapter 6
Taking TCM to the ER

About half way into the school year at ACTCM, we began learning tongue and pulse diagnosis. Of the two, tongue diagnosis was easier than pulse diagnosis.

Tongue Diagnosis

We looked at the tongue size, shape, color, and texture. Any motion, such as quivering, and the appearance of the tongue coating are also important aspects of the examination. A Western physician looks at the tongue merely for signs of dehydration, anemia, and perhaps fungal infections. In TCM, a discipline that uses no invasive techniques, observation of the tongue plays a far greater role in diagnosis. For the TCM practitioner, it is a window to the internal condition of the body.

I was amazed at all the clues tongue diagnosis offered the clinician. From the size and shape, one could diagnose not only dehydration but also fluid retention or edema. Tongue color is very important. As in Western diagnosis, pallor means anemia. In TCM, an excessively dark red color also has significance—it is a sign of either organ congestion or Heat. A yellowish coating signifies an infectious or inflammatory state. A thick wet coating often signifies a dysfunction in digestion.

TCM includes in its paradigm a system like reflexology in which different organs of the body have their representative locations on the tongue. The same applies to the French Ear Acupuncture system and the Korean Hand Acupuncture system. Discoloration, such as a dark spot, on a certain area of the tongue might signify a disease in the represented area of the body. As I became more proficient, I was even able to find signs of past surgery in the lines and indentations of the tongue.

Pulse Diagnosis

We were also taught to feel the pulses at the wrist. In addition to noting the rate and rhythm of the pulse, already familiar from my Western training, we were taught to note the quality of the pulse. We felt the pulse in three locations along about an inch and a half length of the radial artery at the wrist, using our right hand for the patient's right wrist and our left for the patient's left wrist. We felt with index, middle, and ring fingers respectively. Changes in the quality of the pulse at a particular location on the wrist reflect changes in the corresponding body zone. The location of the index finger corresponded to the Upper Burner, the middle finger to the Middle Burner, and the ring finger to the Lower Burner (see chapter 2).

Pulse diagnosis has always intrigued me. Diagnosing an ailment by the quality of the pulse took on meaning as I correlated these qualities with Western physiology. A slippery 滑 pulse is one in which the pulse wave seems to begin before the previous one has a chance to fall all the way to baseline. TCM practitioners often take pride in their ability to diagnose early pregnancy. A pregnant woman will typically have a slippery pulse because during pregnancy, there is a marked increase in blood volume and cardiac output, accounting for the characteristic change.

When a patient is stressed or in pain, he has a wiry 引 or Liver-type pulse, indicative of blood vessel constriction. The description of Liver-type pulse validated my interpretation of the TCM Liver being the sympathetic nervous system. With stress or pain, the sympathetic nervous system acts by constricting the blood vessels, causing them to feel wiry.

When the body mounts an immune response and blood rushes to the part of body being attacked, the pulse to that region of the body becomes floating 浮. The pulse is close to the surface, and it seems to float up to meet the examiner's finger. The explanation is that with infection or inflammation, the blood vessels in the affected area dilate, bringing the needed immune cells to do battle in defense of that body zone.

For many years I had wondered how, by feeling the pulse at three locations on the wrist, TCM physicians were able to correlate what they found with the three zones of the body. One day, the explanation dawned on me. As the heart pumps blood into the main blood vessel, the aorta, its branching vessels send blood to various parts of the body. With each heartbeat, there is a series of waves along the radial artery, or any blood vessel for that matter. The first wave is from the initial branches sending blood to the brain, heart, and lungs. The second wave is from branches sending blood to the visceral organs, and the third and last is from branches to the urogenital region and lower limbs in sequential order. Feeling the three great waves created in the blood flow along the length of the radial artery, the Chinese physicians could determine the condition of the three zones of the body. Pulse diagnosis required sensitivity and skill. I seized every available opportunity to practice on any willing subject.

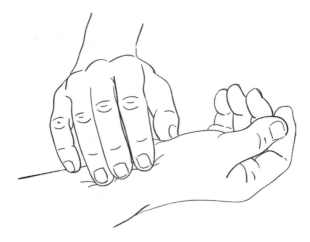

Fig. 3. Pulse Taking. The examiner's three fingers are, with each pulsation, palpating the three waves, representing the three body zones.

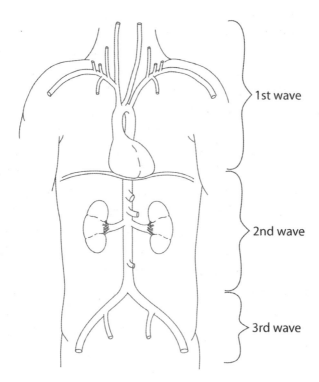

1st wave

2nd wave

3rd wave

Fig. 4. The Three Great Waves of the Chinese Pulse.

The ER: My Virtual Lab

While I was attending ACTCM, I continued to work in the emergency room. The ER became my virtual laboratory. I tried to apply what I had learned in the evenings and weekends to various situations at work. My subjects were roughly divided into two groups. Those in the horizontal group were patients wheeled in on gurneys; those in the vertical group were the ER staff, who, when there was a lull at work, would describe their symptoms to me, asking for my TCM diagnosis. As I applied TCM to the ER scene, I began to sort out which conditions were candidates for the Eastern approach and which were not.

For the ER patients who were brought in comatose, once they were given the appropriate Western emergency care, I tried the Chinese emergency acupuncture technique of needling them briefly above the upper lip to awaken them from coma. I found this method ineffective. In fact, I found no true medical emergencies in which I could apply the TCM treatments I had learned. If patients required intravenous fluids or drugs, the Eastern way of brewing herbs just could not compare to rapid Western methods.

On the other hand, as I used my newly learned tongue and pulse diagnosis to see how "balanced" the ER staff was, I discovered almost all of them had, by TCM standards, some abnormalities. Some were symptomatic, others were not. Paula had recently given birth to twins and returned to work on the evening shift as a ward clerk after only a short maternity leave. Although she had no symptoms, her tongue showed signs of Spleen Deficiency, indicating that her immune system was weakened. Darlene, a nurse, had a skin cancer taken out of her leg and, shortly thereafter, had a miscarriage. Her pulses and tongue showed Blood Deficiency, indicating that her body had not totally made up for the blood loss from her miscarriage. From the TCM perspective, it was rare to find anyone completely normal. Yet they were all well enough to be working in the ER. I wondered if they were walking time bombs.

Disease Stages

I began to realize that every disease progresses in stages. Generally, a disease begins with certain imbalances, barely detectable, and only later does it become symptomatic. The duration of the stages varies depending on the disease. In an acute infection, the stages are short. A patient with strep throat will develop fever and painful swallowing in a matter of hours. With other diseases, like cancer or heart disease, the early stage might last for years. Eastern medicine works best in the early stages of a disease because it can help reverse the imbalances in the host and promote self-healing. It can also be effective in the intermediate stage, when there are symptoms. In advanced stages, TCM methods of working on imbalances in the host are no longer enough. At this point, a Western approach should be chosen. After the critical problem is taken care of with a Western approach, Eastern medicine may again have a role during the recovery period.

Some skeptics explain the popularity of complementary medicine by saying that the patients who feel helped by it were actually not that sick and that it is the practitioner's attentiveness rather than the treatment that made the patient feel better. From the Western perspective, that may appear to be. Complementary care practitioners do spend more time with patients and go into detail getting their history. The patients seeking this kind of care are not severely ill, but they usually have problems that do not seem to completely resolve using Western methods. Nevertheless, their problems are real and not just imagined. Success with using Eastern treatments is also real and not just a placebo effect. Western skeptics try to explain it away because they do not understand the paradigm. The difference between Western medicine and TCM is that TCM diagnosis focuses not just on disease but also on the person's own ability to fight disease. This entails detailed history taking. Although they lack specificity, pulse and tongue diagnosis are extremely sensitive tools. Sometimes they can pick up diseases before symptoms appear. Often they can detect deficiencies in the patient's ability to heal and work on improving the host's recovery. The West has an aphorism: "If it isn't broken, don't fix it." TCM may be able to detect small cracks and mend them before they actually break.

The sensitivity of TCM diagnosis became apparent to me during the course of treating a physician's wife with acupuncture for a musculoskeletal condition. As I was contemplating giving her herbs for another problem she had, I happened to feel her pulses. The lung position pulse was floating, a sign that the body is mounting an immune response, typical in the early stage of a viral infection. At the end of the session my patient said, "I'll see you next week." "No," I told her, "you are probably coming down with the flu, and I shall probably see you in two weeks." After two weeks, she returned. She had indeed come down with the flu. Her husband was amazed at my prescience. Actually, it was a simple diagnosis to make using TCM methods.

I used to think that the only treatment for acute appendicitis was surgery. When my teacher, Dr. Lai, told me that he had treated a man for appendicitis by using acupuncture, I was skeptical. The patient had been experiencing pain in the lower right region of his abdomen, and my teacher had acupunctured him until the pain was relieved. This cannot be true, I thought. Perhaps the diagnosis of appendicitis was in error. There are abdominal pains that could mimic appendicitis. The only absolute proof is when a surgeon operates and can actually see the inflamed appendix. As I look back with the perspective that diseases evolve in stages, and I think about how appendicitis develops, the account of my teacher's treatment becomes more plausible.

The appendix is a small worm-like tube branching out from the intestines. It is situated at the junction of the small and large intestine. If stool passing down to be eliminated is hard, sometimes a small stone-like piece, called a fecolith, will be stuck at the opening of the appendix, thereby blocking it. At this stage, if there is no intervention, the appendix wall becomes inflamed and swollen, worsening the obstruction. The secretions of the appendix, which normally empty into the large intestine, have nowhere to go and therefore stagnate and become infected. The appendix becomes a closed tube containing infected fluid whose volume continually increases. If there is no intervention, the appendix will eventually rupture. Before that happens, surgery is needed. At the early stage, when the fecolith is just beginning to block the opening of the appendix, intervention with acupuncture could work. If the smooth muscles of the appendix wall could be relaxed and allowed to dilate, then the opening might become wide enough to let the fecolith pass into the large intestine. Acupuncture and some herbs can act to relax the smooth muscle and dilate the wall of the appendix, stopping the progression to appendicitis.

In my dual role as both TCM student and ER physician, I observed a certain pattern of events. Often, patients who came to the ER with an acute catastrophic condition had undergone a recent invasive Western procedure. Two cases come to mind. One was an older man who had had recent cataract surgery and was brought to the ER with a stroke. Another case was a young boy who had had dental surgery the day before and came in with acute appendicitis. Later on in my practice, I observed other similar cases.

I began to realize that the "walking well" have a certain balance that we in Western medicine call homeostasis, the intrinsic ability of the body to keep itself in equilibrium. For some, like the older man, homeostasis might have been tenuous, and the balance was tipped by the stress of the surgery. Although cataract surgery is not considered a major operation, we know that with any surgery, the body usually mobilizes its clotting mechanisms to prepare for blood loss. In a man whose arteries to the brain were already narrowed, that extra increase in the blood clotting function might have been enough to tip the balance and cause his stroke.

As for the young boy with appendicitis, I could see how his disease evolved. The codeine his dentist prescribed for pain made him constipated. Because his mouth hurt, he probably did not drink enough fluids, and this caused dehydration. Constipation and dehydration led to fecolith formation, which then progressed to appendicitis.

When I was a first-year anesthesiology resident at Columbia Presbyterian Hospital, we used to have rounds (mini-conferences) in which dramatic cases were discussed. There was a plethora of these cases characterized by near-disaster and rescue among the trainees. One of our attending physicians remarked, "My days are rather dull. I never seem to encounter all this drama you people report." His comment made me think about what distinguished him, a seasoned anesthesiologist, from us, the neophytes. The experienced, competent anesthesiologist anticipates disaster and takes measures to avert it before it happens. The measure of a good doctor should not be how many dramatic rescues he performs on his patients but how stable and "not sick" he can keep them.

In addition to detecting early stages of disease, TCM has a role in treating conditions of a chronic nature. Western medicine often reaches an impasse when treating certain people whose conditions plateau. In these cases, Eastern medicine plays a significant role. By infusing energy with herbs, or improving blood flow to a diseased area using acupuncture, the body can be induced to heal itself.

One day while working a shift in the emergency room, I bumped into Bill, an ER orderly, in the hospital corridor. He told me he had missed nearly three weeks of work because of a painful condition. His affliction was epididymitis, which is an inflammation of the tube around the testicle. Despite being on nonsteroidal anti-inflammatory drugs and the second course of antibiotics prescribed by his urologist, he was no better. After consulting with my teacher, Dr. Lai, I offered to treat Bill with acupuncture and herbs. Since he seemed to have reached an impasse with Western treatments, Bill agreed to try.

I began with acupuncture. Bill was palpably anxious. He watched my every move as I needled (no, I did not needle the organ, but close to it) along the pubic area and inner thigh. Because he had confidence in my competence as an ER physician, he gritted his teeth and was willing to let me continue. I hooked up the needles to the electrical machine Aunt Teresa had given me. (This time I remembered to turn the dials the Chinese way.) At the end of the twenty-minute treatment, Bill arose from the stretcher and looked a bit puzzled. He said, "The pain isn't there anymore. Is it supposed to go away right away?" "I don't know, this is the first time I've done this," I answered. The next day was my day off. I called the emergency room to find out how Bill was. They said he was back at work. He never required any further treatment. Imagine, with the best modern medicine had to offer, this man suffered for weeks and lost time at work from his illness. Then with an ancient remedy consisting of a few needles hooked up to electricity, he was cured in a matter of twenty minutes. The implications were tremendous. More than ever, I was convinced there was validity to TCM.

Being a female in a male-dominated field, I am often mistaken for a nurse. One patient referred to me as "that nurse" when I was training in intensive care. I assumed it was the usual mistake because of my gender. When the nurse told her I was the doctor, the patient said, "I know, but sometimes she's a nurse, too." I considered that a compliment. Over the years, I have found that nurses in general are very receptive to Eastern medicine. Unlike the doctor, who pops in once or twice a day for a matter of minutes to see the patient in the hospital, nurses have ongoing contact with their patients daily. They are often more in touch with how patients feel than doctors are. One ER nurse told me she was enthusiastic about my studying Eastern medicine, saying, "I bet it will make you an even better doctor." I think she was right.

Chapter 7
Fundamental TCM
Treatment Principles

D r. Lai began teaching at ACTCM toward the latter half of the year when we had finished studying theory and moved on to application. Even though his English was barely intelligible, it was evident to everyone that he was an exceptional TCM clinician. Dr. Lai was in his early thirties, and it was amazing that such a youthful Chinese doctor had the depth of knowledge and experience usually seen only in much older individuals. In fact, many patients meeting Dr. Lai for the first time mistook him for the son of the esteemed doctor.

He was born in Canton in 1947. With the Communist takeover of China in 1949, Dr. Lai was stranded in Canton with his grandmother while his parents were in Hong Kong. When he turned twelve, his grandmother became ill. Fate dictated that he grow up quickly since he bore the responsibility of taking his grandmother to see doctors. While seeking a cure for her illness, he developed a keen interest in medicine. Concurrently, the political upheaval leading to the disastrous Cultural Revolution was brewing. By the time he was fifteen, the Cultural Revolution brought Dr. Lai's formal schooling to an abrupt halt. From then on, he began a program of self-education in medicine. He bought books, studied in libraries, and sought out practical training from noted TCM practitioners. He applied what he learned by treating the sick and poor in surrounding villages. Often he had to devise treatments from the limited resources at hand. In 1970, at the age of twenty-three, he made his escape from China, swimming across the short stretch of water between Canton and Hong Kong. Two years later, he immigrated to the United States and helped his entire family to immigrate. By the time he was thirty-four and teaching at ACTCM, he already had twenty years of clinical experience.

I was one of a handful of students to whom Dr. Lai extended an open invitation to observe how he treated patients in his office. This was the opportunity of a lifetime. There was just one glitch. Since I am Cantonese, Dr. Lai preferred speaking to me in Cantonese, but my vocabulary was that of a grade school student. I understood only about 60 percent of what he said. Now I really regretted my inattention in Chinese school. Remembering how to say "The little cat jumped and jumped and jumped" from Book One, Lesson One was just not enough.

In addition to the Chinese language barrier, there was also the TCM language barrier. When Dr. Lai explained, "Now this is a Lung disease, and we know we have to calm the Liver and support the Spleen to help the Lung," I would say to myself, What in the world do the liver and spleen have to do with treating the lung? I just nodded deferentially. When Dr. Lai used his broken English to explain disease processes and treatment principles, using TCM terminology, to his Caucasian patients, it was obvious that they could not understand a word of what he said either. They too nodded deferentially.

The pungent smell of herbs permeated Dr. Lai's office—his wife packaged uncooked ones for some patients and boiled some on a hot plate for other patients who needed this service. On the walls hung plaques given by grateful patients extolling his abilities as a healer. The waiting room also served as the pharmacy. Patients sat waiting either to be seen or to pick up the herb prescription being filled by Mrs. Lai after the doctor had seen them. As Mrs. Lai filled prescriptions, friends and family would drop in to chat, giving the office a mom-and-pop family atmosphere.

Cubicles, just large enough for an acupuncture table and a portable electric heater, made up his treatment rooms. For privacy, a curtain separated the entry to each cubicle from the hallway. A large desk sat in the center of the consultation room. On the desk was a little pillow on which patients could rest their wrist for pulse taking. A blood pressure apparatus sat alongside the pillow, bespeaking Dr. Lai's openness to Western medicine. A bookcase stood behind the desk where, among other books, there was a Chinese-English medical dictionary, which I found of immense help when communicating with Dr. Lai.

Other objects on the bookcase were evidence of Dr. Lai's syncretism. A statue of Kwan-Yin, the Chinese goddess of mercy, stood on the top shelf, a statue of Christian praying hands graced the shelf below Kwan-Yin, and an "I'm for Nixon" campaign button was propped against the praying hands. As a boy, Dr. Lai had been quite ill. He had prayed to Kwan-Yin, and was healed. Although he could not accept that Jesus was the only way to salvation, he considered Jesus Christ too great not to be acknowledged. "What about Nixon?" I asked. "It was Nixon's immigration policy that allowed refugees from Communist China to come to the United States," he answered. This enabled him to immigrate in 1972.

Dr. Lai has an ebullient personality. He is a man with a big voice and a big heart. I have seen him waive fees for some patients who were in financial straits and take the same patients out to dinner on their birthdays. He loved to converse about a wide range of topics: medicine, philosophy, world affairs, and the economy, to name a few. Often deep in discussion, he would be oblivious of the time. His wife would have to run into the consultation room to remind him there were patients waiting. Unusual for a TCM practitioner, he is very receptive to Western medicine and reads extensively about it. He is not opposed to surgery or cancer chemotherapy but works with patients to supplement their Western treatment with herbal therapy. In the spirit of Louis Pasteur, Dr. Lai is a pioneer. He experimented with herbs, using himself as the test subject.

Dr. Lai's clinical acumen is uncanny. Once when he was treating a patient with a stroke that had left the patient's body half paralyzed, he asked me to order a test to check for the carotid artery blood flow to the part of the brain controlling the non-paralyzed side. From his pulse diagnosis, he determined that this artery was blocked. Indeed, the carotid ultrasound showed critical narrowing of the carotid artery on the side Dr. Lai had suspected.

A woman saw him for chronic upper back and chest pain that, despite myriad testing, had defied Western diagnosis. Dr. Lai sat at his desk, looked at the patient, and saw that one collarbone was higher than the other. With that observation, he was able to diagnose that the cause of her pain was a misalignment in her upper back, which he treated with acupuncture; her pain resolved.

Whenever I visited his office, Dr. Lai had me sit at the desk with him, and he introduced me to each patient. The English-speaking patients appreciated my presence. I served as interpreter, not only of the language, but also of any lab or X-ray results they brought to the office. On each patient, he would point out the subtle nuances in the feeling of the pulse and the appearance of the tongue to me. Next, he would teach the TCM diagnosis and then the treatment principle. Finally, with lightning speed, he wrote out his herbal prescription, using cursive script that only his wife could read, while simultaneously naming the herbs aloud. When it came to illegible handwriting, Western doctors had nothing on Dr. Lai. I had to take notes at a breakneck pace. Since he named the herbs in Chinese, I developed my own phonetic shorthand to keep up. Gradually I learned to write the Chinese characters for the herbs.

Despite his profound grasp of TCM, Dr. Lai also avidly read Chinese translations of Western medical literature. A woman who had suffered from infertility, on becoming pregnant after receiving TCM treatments, asked him about all the dos and don'ts during her pregnancy. He went on and on with advice, which sounded to me like Chinese folklore, such as, "Avoid going to the zoo so that your baby won't come out looking like a monkey." Then she asked, "What should I do to make sure my baby is smart?" He answered, "Oh, that's in the genes, nothing you can do about that."

Support the Host as well as Fight the Invader

In late 1981, when I began studying with Dr. Lai, the HIV-AIDS epidemic, which at the time still lacked a name, was underway in the United States. Often, desperately sick people who had exhausted Western methods came to seek his help. I had the opportunity to see exotic cases I had only read about in medical texts. It was in this setting that I learned the essential TCM treatment principle: when treating a foreign invader such as a virus or bacteria, use not only cleansing herbs, comparable to the Western antibiotic or antiviral, aimed at destroying the invader, but simultaneously support the host's own ability to fight the invader with immune-boosting herbs. Early in the HIV-AIDS epidemic, before antiretroviral drugs were developed, what Western doctors learned was that no matter how potent the drugs, if the host immune system was nonfunctioning, recovery was hopeless. Since the HIV-AIDS epidemic, Western medicine began exploring the concept of immune modulation, a concept that has long been part of TCM.

The same principle applied to building up a host's defense mechanisms when treating cancer patients. For these people, during radiation and chemotherapy, Dr. Lai would use herbs to treat the side effects, such as bone marrow depression, nausea, and fatigue. When the radiation and chemotherapy sessions ended, he would begin treatments with cleansing, anti-cancer type herbs, which he balanced with immune-boosting herbs. Finding the appropriate balance, the proportion of cleansing to tonifying herbs for a particular patient, is the challenge every TCM practitioner faces. To gain mastery over this art was my goal as Dr. Lai's student and mentee.

Economics of Energy

The concept I call the economics of energy is key in the TCM approach to understanding health and disease. Dr. Lai used a metaphor to explain it: "You have only so much money in the bank, and you can't keep spending more than you have." Each one of us has a finite supply of energy. When the energy is adequate for all our bodily requirements, we remain healthy. When extra demand is put on our bodies from various causes such as stress, infection, trauma, lack of sleep, or change in diet, sometimes supply cannot keep up with demand, and the weakest link gives way.

A research study into the effects of increasing the temperature in operating rooms demonstrates this principle (Kurz, et al. 1996). Customarily, operating room temperatures are kept cool for the comfort of the surgical team clad in their head-to-foot attire while working under bright lights. The study investigated the effects of warming up the operating room a few degrees. They found that the increase in temperature resulted in faster wound healing, fewer wound infections, and earlier hospital discharge for the patients. Researchers explained their findings this way: With colder temperatures, the blood vessels to the operative site tend to constrict in order to preserve body temperature. With decreased blood flow, fewer infection-fighting white blood cells were carried to the surgical wound, and this led to more wound infections. With the economics of energy, we can explain the phenomenon this way: with a warmer operating room, the energy usually expended by the patient to keep warm was conserved and could then be directed to wound healing.

Why do we catch more colds and flu in winter months? The Western scientific explanation is that with cold weather, the blood vessels in our noses constrict, and therefore fewer germ-fighting cells and antibodies are available to fight viruses. The Chinese ancients explained colds by attributing them to the Cold evil. Economics of energy could explain the seasonal tendency this way: in cold weather, more of our energy is expended on keeping us warm at the expense of fighting viruses.

Dr. Lai taught that acupuncture redistributes energy but does not increase it. Acupuncture increases blood flow to the diseased area being needled. If the components that promote healing carried in the blood are inadequate, or the overall blood supply is low, acupuncture may not improve the patient's condition. Patients with inadequate energy need to have their energy replenished with herbs for acupuncture to be effective. In my practice, I found this principle often applied to the elderly who had multiple medical problems. For the same malady, acupuncture might be effective for a young healthy patient but ineffective for a debilitated elderly patient.

A compounding factor in patients with low energy was inadequate protein in the diet, often seen among vegetarians. Dr. Lai advised such patients to gradually reintroduce meat into their diets. He said that a vegetarian diet was adequate to meet the body's energy demands only if one was leading a monk's life, with minimal mental and physical stress. He shook his head over Americans who, while living in the horn of plenty, chose to adopt the lifestyle of those living in a third world country.

At an orphanage in Taiwan, a missionary nurse once told me about abandoned children whose bodies were covered with skin sores. In spite of meticulous wound care, the children's sores did not resolve until they were fed a normal diet adequate in protein. I personally have counseled vegetarian patients to reintroduce meat, fish, or poultry into their diets and have watched such symptoms as rashes resolve without further therapy.

When inordinate demands are placed on the body, it tends to divert energy from one area to another, robbing Peter to pay Paul. May was a woman in her early forties who came to me complaining of chronic intestinal upset, poor digestion, and gassiness. Since Western medications had not worked for her, I decided to use herbal therapy. Over the course of treatment for her intestinal problem, I noticed that May's face developed a glow. She and her husband had been married for twenty years and were infertile. After so many years, they had accepted the fact that they would be childless. When May told me about her missed period, I tested her for pregnancy, and her test came back positive. She went on to deliver a beautiful baby boy.

May's case demonstrates the economics of energy. May's reproductive system was most likely weak to begin with. Her digestive problem diverted energy to the digestive system and away from her reproductive system, robbing it of the needed energy to conceive. When her digestive disorder resolved, her body's energy was channeled back to the reproductive system. After May's case, whenever I treated infertility with herbs or acupuncture, instead of focusing obsessively on the fertility issue, I advised patients that the herbs would simply improve their health. If they became pregnant, it would be a bonus. My approach definitely proved less draining for patients both emotionally and financially when compared to fertility clinics, and it often succeeded!

Finding the Ben 本

The key to both Eastern and Western medicine is accurate diagnosis. But for TCM, diagnosing the disease is only the first step. The disease is called the Biao 表. It is the external manifestation of the patient's root problem. Treatment of the Biao, while important, is not enough. The TCM physician needs to determine the Ben, or root problem, the basic imbalance in the patient that caused him to lose his ability to fend off disease in the first place.

Interestingly, the Chinese character for Ben is a tree (木) with its roots (本) extending below the surface of the earth. You need to dig below the surface to find the root. If the Ben is not addressed, the condition might not completely resolve. If addressed, the doctor puts the patient's body "back on its feet," so to speak. The key to identifying the imbalance is correct diagnosis.

One of my patients, Winnie, returned to work shortly after giving birth to her baby. She developed a recalcitrant, itchy rash. Despite many visits to the dermatologist and multiple applications of various topical steroids, the rash persisted. It would temporarily resolve with the creams, only to return once Winnie stopped applying them. Finally, I treated Winnie using tonifying (enhancing) Blood 補血 and Kidney Qi 腎氣 herbs. According to TCM teaching, these two areas become depleted after a mother gives birth to her baby. With my treatments, the rash completely resolved. For Winnie, the rash was the Biao, the outward manifestation of her condition. The Ben, or root problem, was depleted Blood and Kidney Qi because of her postpartum state and early resumption of work. The phenomenon of postpartum patients developing various new maladies was so common in my practice that there were times I considered labeling it the postpartum syndrome. I have been able to help many other postpartum patients like Winnie who developed different Biao conditions after giving birth.

Tonify the Deficient 補虛

The TCM word "Bu 補" is translated "to tonify." The word, which has a radical on the left for clothing, actually means "to mend." In Chinese, if you have a tear in your clothing, you mend it, using this word. If you have a cavity in a tooth, Bu 補 is used to mean filling the cavity. If there is a defect in a road, this same word is used to mean repairing the defect. In TCM, when the doctor diagnoses a deficiency, the Chinese word "Bu 補" describes what the doctor prescribes to replenish the deficient entity.

When a bodily function is weak, TCM practitioners call it deficient-organ Qi 內臟氣虛 and prescribe herbs to tonify 補 or strengthen the function. For instance, if Kidney Qi is deficient 腎氣虛, the Chinese practitioner uses Kidney tonifying herbs 補腎藥, which work by improving blood flow to that weakened TCM organ. When other entities, such as blood or other fluids, are deficient, the practitioner will use tonifying herbs to help replenish them.

Regarding tonifying Blood herbs 補血藥, I asked Dr. Lai if they stimulate red blood cell production by the bone marrow, comparable to Erythropoietin, the drug commonly used for anemia caused by chemotherapy. He said that stimulating production might be only one aspect of tonifying Blood. We know that red blood cells have an average life span of 120 days. In addition to stimulating production of new red blood cells, Blood tonifying herbs may rejuvenate old red blood cells to function a bit longer until the newly produced red cells mature.

Tonifying Yin 補陰 fluid is a concept unique to TCM. This process does not simply mean hydration or increasing fluid intake. It involves improving the function of various glands that produce body fluids, such as the mucous, saliva, and digestive glands. The mechanism may be twofold: through dilating the glands' ducts and through improving blood flow to the glands.

Dr. Lai pointed out that sometimes both Yin and Yang energy can be depleted. If one is more depleted than the other, the patient can appear to have a deficiency in the more depleted one only. In these cases, you have to tonify both Yin and Yang to restore normality. Perhaps this explains why some Chinese patients say they are deficient but cannot tolerate being tonified 虛不受補. To them, Bu 補 or tonifying herbs are synonymous with Yang tonification 補陽 herbs. When solely Yang tonification 補陽 is used in patients with dual deficiencies, they end up with symptoms of relative Yang excess such as dry mouth and constipation because the need to tonify their Yin deficiency was overlooked.

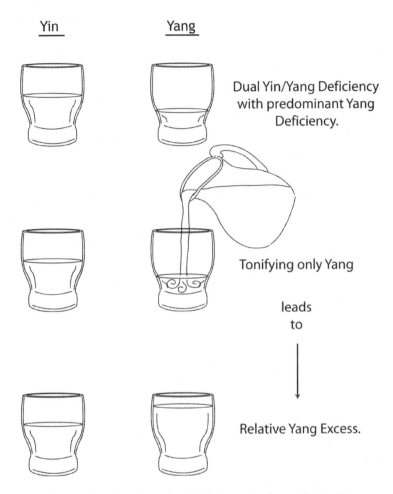

Yin   Yang

Dual Yin/Yang Deficiency
with predominant Yang
Deficiency.

Tonifying only Yang

leads
to

Relative Yang Excess.

Fig. 5. Tonifying Yang alone in a dual deficiency leads to relative Yang excess.

Fannie was in her forties when she developed the autoimmune disease Sjogren's syndrome, characterized by dryness throughout the body. Western medicine's explanation for Sjogren's syndrome is that the body inappropriately makes antibodies that attack all its fluid-secreting glands. Fannie had a beautiful singing voice and sang in the church choir. Now, with dry eyes and a dry mouth, she could barely talk. Her digestive juices were diminished, causing poor appetite and constipation.

Her deficiencies were complex. She lacked not only Yin fluid but also Yang function in the form of immune energy. Treatment was tricky. Restoring both Yin and Yang were involved. I referred Fannie to Dr. Lai. In addition to tonifying Yin, her major problem, he also tonified Stomach and Spleen. Her decreased ability to secrete fluids meant Fannie's digestive tract functioned poorly. On top of that, her weak immune system, which was what led to her body's attack on its own glands in the first place, needed to be strengthened. Spleen herbs help these two problems, but Spleen herbs tend to be drying. Dr. Lai prescribed a preponderance of Yin tonifying herbs relative to the Spleen herbs. Under his care, her singing voice was restored, and she once again sang in the church choir.

I discovered that the Chinese often have a distorted view of Bu 補. They think that using tonifying herbs will fortify them, even if they are not in a deficient state. My understanding of the concept is that you tonify only where there is a deficiency. Dr. Lai agreed. "You don't sew a patch on a new suit," he said. My Chinese patients frequently asked me to recommend a brand of vitamins for them. I used to think their request silly. My usual answer was, "It doesn't matter, any multivitamin will do. Chances are you might not even need them, but they won't hurt." It finally dawned on me that they actually thought vitamins were equivalent to TCM tonifying or Bu 補 herbs. When I told these patients that vitamins are not the same as Bu 補 herbs, their eyes would light up as if to say, "Really?" Since then, I made sure to include this bit of information when giving health lectures to Chinese audiences. Many have come up to me afterwards to thank me because that was the first time they heard their misconception explained.

The Herbal Prescription

For years, with the exception of treating serious infection or cancer, Western medicine believed in monotherapy: one drug for one disease whenever possible. For treating hypertension, for instance, you titrate the dosage of one drug and add a second drug only if the condition remains uncontrolled on maximum doses of the first drug. Recently, Western drug therapy has evolved into poly-pharmacy. This is the usage of multiple drugs to treat one condition in order to get a synergistic effect and minimize side effects. TCM's approach has always been polypharmacy, using multiple herbs to treat a condition. Dr. Lai taught me to choose three or four herbs from a category that addressed the main condition. These were the major herbs. The other elements of the prescription consisted of herbs to balance the side effects of the major herbs, herbs to enhance absorption, herbs to address any accompanying symptoms, and herbs to correct the imbalances in the host and restore energy.

A typical herb prescription for the common cold or flu consists of cold-cleansing herbs to fight the virus, lowering-Qi herbs to stop coughing, herbs to reduce and break up phlegm, moistening lung Yin herbs to thin secretions, and energy herbs to boost the host's immunity.

The Confluence of East and West

There were times in the early 1980s when what Dr. Lai said seemed to contradict what I had learned in my Western training. Time proved him right. He told me infections had to be treated with a full course of herbs to guard against future arthritis. At the time, I thought the idea was most likely a holdover from the days before penicillin, when rheumatic fever with its migratory arthritis was a common complication of streptococcal infection. In California, where streptococcal infections are promptly treated with antibiot-ics, one can hardly find any cases of rheumatic fever. Interestingly though, Western medicine has found links between arthritis and past infections, such as certain infectious diarrhea. It is called "reactive arthritis," something Dr. Lai described long ago.

Dr. Lai recommended treating stomach ulcers as if they were an infection and told me that stomach ulcers could progress to cancer. At that time, the early 1980s, Western medicine taught that gastric ulcers were either benign or malignant. You rarely worried about a benign ulcer becoming malignant. The standard treatment for stomach ulcers was H-2 blockers such as cimetidine to discourage acid secretion by the stomach. No one felt that ulcers were caused by infections. Now it is an established fact that ulcers are frequently caused by infection with the bacterium H. Pylori, and that there is a link between this bacterium and a form of stomach cancer. Today, if there is evidence of H. Pylori infection in an ulcer patient, we treat with a course of two antibiotics and an agent to discourage stomach acid secretion.

In the early 1990s, I saw a patient who presented atypical symptoms of a heart attack. Her pain was confined to her throat. When I examined her throat, I found it was normal, but her tongue had a thick yellowish coating, which, according to TCM, is a sign of Heat, signifying inflammation or infection. The EKG definitely showed an acute heart attack as the cause of her throat pain. The case was puzzling to me. The patient had a heart attack caused by a blockage of one or more coronary arteries. She had no infection that I could find. Yet using my TCM examination, I found signs suggestive of infection or inflammation. Dr. Lai told me that in his experience, this finding of Heat or inflammation was usual in coronary heart disease. Now, Western studies show that inflammation is an important factor in coronary occlusion and that there is sometimes even a link between coronary occlusion and certain infections such as Chlamydia (Buffon, et al. 2002; Wierzbicki and Hagmeyer 2000). Long ago, Dr. Lai had already linked inflammation with heart disease. The sensitivity of the TCM method in the hands of an astute clinician proved a powerful tool.

While working with Dr. Lai, I sensed that as long as he was available, problems would find a solution. Whenever I stepped into his office, I felt, as did the patients, a sense of security and optimism. Knowing him gave me the courage to embark on my practice of integrating Eastern and Western medicine in the early 1980s, when it was still an unmapped frontier.

"First do no harm"

— GALEN

Chapter 8

New Beginnings: Starting an Integrated Practice

At ACTCM, I selected classes pertinent to my needs and interests. With my background, I felt free to skip classes such as basic anatomy and physiology. By early 1982, after a year of formal classes at ACTCM on herbology and acupuncture and my practicum with Dr. Lai, I quit work in the ER and launched an integrated practice of Western and Eastern medicine. I envisioned my practice to be a virtual Utopia for patients, especially for those in the Chinese community. Up to then, these patients had to triage themselves as to which practitioner, Eastern or Western, to see for their ailments. There was no communication between practitioners of these respective disciplines. If the Eastern practitioner prescribed herbs, patients had to decide for themselves whether to discontinue any drugs prescribed by their Western physicians. Such important decisions were made based on tradition or advice from well-meaning but untrained friends and family. I, as someone trained in both disciplines, would be able to offer them the best of both worlds under one roof. My Utopian vision turned out to be a fantasy. It turned out that my Chinese patients expected only

Western medical care from me. If they wanted herbs or acupuncture, they would see their own TCM doctors.

Before opening my dual practice, I sought the advice of Western colleagues who were already using acupuncture in their practices. At that time there was only a handful. One colleague told me that his strategy was to practice the best Western medicine he knew to first gain the acceptance and credulity of his Western colleagues. I became very aware of his sage advice. I remembered how, in medical school, we were indoctrinated to view any disciplines outside of allopathic medicine with condescension. As an intern, I was appalled to hear from an acquaintance who was a world-class ice skater that she was seeing a chiropractor.

When I was working in emergency medicine, John, one of the ER orderlies, came to work with a crick in his neck. The ER staff went to work on John using traction, heat, ultrasound, and injections of Valium and Demerol. Despite all these measures, they could not straighten his neck out. Then one ER colleague thought of trying a chiropractor. We looked in the yellow pages and sent John to a nearby school of chiropractic. After one treatment, he was much better and able to hold his head straight. This experience taught me humility. It also taught me prudence.

My practice began on a small scale. I time-shared an office with an established internist, Ed. I had professional cards printed, indicating I did family practice and acupuncture. I did not mention Chinese herbal therapy on my card. I felt publicizing that aspect of my practice would invite criticism. It was common in Western hospitals to implicate Chinese herbs whenever a Chinese patient presented a problem that was difficult to diagnose. This mentality was convenient and required no objective proof. Chinese herbal treatments and herbalists became easy scapegoats. By the 1980s, acupuncture had already earned some acceptance, so being a physician-acupuncturist was less controversial. I remained a closet Chinese herbalist for many years, known only to the patients I treated. Occasionally, word leaked out about my prescribing

Chinese herbs, and I overheard the ridiculing comments some of my colleagues made. I kept up a high standard of Western practice, though, and was therefore able to remain above reproach. I carefully chose to use alternative methods only when Western treatment options had been tried and failed, or when I knew there were no good Western options.

Sometimes I reminisce about the early days in my practice when I was not so busy. Money was scarce, but time was abundant. I had time to sew cloth patient gowns, which I preferred over the stiff, scratchy, disposable paper ones. One patient commented on how comfortable these gowns were, and even inquired as to where she could buy them. I told her that I had them made to order. During my first year, I saw an average of three patients per day. One day, when I was seeing my third and last patient, the receptionist I shared with Ed announced within hearing range of the patient, "Doctor, your next patient called to say he will be a little late." After my third patient left, I queried the receptionist as to who the next patient was. "The patient who just left was your last," she replied, "but I didn't want her to feel lonely."

Using TCM to Treat Asthma

During my studies, my enthusiasm for TCM overflowed to my friends. When I started my integrated practice, one of my very first patients was my friend Betty, a nurse originally from Hong Kong. Betty was in her forties, and she had suffered from severe asthma since the age of nineteen. She had the classic triad of nasal polyps, aspirin allergy, and bronchial asthma. Her condition was so severe that every night she had to prop herself up with several pillows to breathe. When she went to work, she had to take a few puffs of her inhaler before she could negotiate the hill where her hospital was located. On average, Betty required one or two courses of steroids a year when she had acute flares of her asthma.

The herbal prescription for Betty was one of the first I ever wrote. Besides lowering Qi herbs to improve air flow in her bronchial tubes, it included herbs for clearing sputum, tonifying Yin herbs to help her mucous membranes stay moistened, quelling Wind herbs for her allergic rhinitis, tonifying Kidney herbs (a standard ingredient for treating respiratory problems), and tonifying Spleen herbs to boost her weak immune system. When she saw the prescription I wrote, she laughed aloud. The Chinese characters looked as if a child had written them. My Chinese script was so poor that I was embarrassed to use the customary letterhead for my herbal prescriptions. Instead, I wrote them out on a plain sheet of paper. Word got around the local herbal stores that the writer of my prescriptions was a Caucasian trying to learn TCM. Much later, the herbal storekeepers would say that the writer was an American-born Chinese learning TCM. The reality of my impediment hit home later in my career when my blonde and blue-eyed patient, Donna, told me that when she took my Chinese prescription to an herb shop to be filled, the storekeeper commented, "My, you are very smart. You know how to treat yourself and even write Chinese!"

A month after I began treating her with herbs, Betty called one day to say her asthma was very severe. I made a house call, and indeed found that her breathing was quite labored. In addition to giving her an injection of epinephrine as acute intervention, I tried at the same time to treat her with acupuncture. She still required a course of oral steroids. Once her asthma was under control, I tapered her steroids and continued herbs. That was the last time she ever required steroids. Highly motivated, she faithfully continued the herbs I prescribed, and over a period of about three years, her asthma completely disappeared. As time passed, she needed her inhaler less and less, even when she had to climb the hill to work. After three years, she finally was able to stop the nasty tasting herbs and dispense with her inhaler. Her symptoms have never recurred.

On reviewing her chart, I can see that for the first three years while on the herbs, she still came down with asthmatic bronchitis about once or twice a year, but she no longer required steroids. On her annual physical exam four years after starting the herbs, she had no complaints of wheezing. In order to review Betty's chart, I needed to return to the office where I had previously practiced. Her present doctor, who took over my primary practice, said with surprise, "I didn't even know she had asthma."

My approach to Betty's case is typical of how I integrated Eastern and Western treatments. When Betty's asthma was severe and difficult to control, I relied predominantly on Western methods, using TCM treatment as a supplement. After the acute condition was controlled with Western therapy, I continued the TCM therapy while maintaining her simultaneously on Western medication. Gradually, Betty herself recognized that the need for her Western medicine was diminishing and stopped using it. The remarkable aspect of her case is that after three years of TCM treatment, resolution of the problem has been maintained.

Genetics and environment are the two factors influencing health. Each of us is born with a genetic predisposition to certain conditions. In the years before a condition occurs, the body's inner strength, or Qi, seems adequate to stave off the disease. Then, at a certain point, because of factors in either the internal or external environment, that mechanism decompensates, and the condition becomes manifested. In Betty's case, this decompensation occurred at the age of nineteen when she began suffering from asthma. The precipitating factors may have been the stress of adjusting to a new country and studying for her future career. TCM's treatment goal is to restore the body's own homeostatic balance to the pre-morbid state. With this approach, the disease resolution is more lasting. At present, I think Betty's predisposition for asthma still exists, and at some time, another stressor could trigger asthma. So far, this has not occurred.

Treating the Ben 本

When patients with multiple problems came to see me for herbal therapy, I faced a logistical problem. How could I prescribe herbs for each and every problem? The total number of herbs required couldn't fit into the pot to be boiled. I subsequently made a remarkable discovery: If I treated the primary problem, or what TCM calls the Ben 本, the accompanying disorders seemed to resolve spontaneously.

A Case of Eczema

Cynthia suffered from severe asthma and eczema. She arrived at my office wheezing and scratching. It was evident that there was a limit as to how many herbs I could prescribe, and I could not address all her problems at once. With that in mind, I began with herbs directed at the most troublesome condition, the asthma. I planned to phase in herbs for the skin after her asthma improved to the point where I could reduce the number of asthma herbs. To my surprise, I found that when Cynthia's asthma resolved, her eczema also cleared. The Western approach would be to treat Cynthia's asthma with inhaled bronchodilators and her eczema with topical steroids, as two separate problems. Actually, both conditions were Biao 表, or external manifestations, of the Ben 本, or root problem, a weakened immune system. When I treated her asthma, Cynthia's prescription contained herbs for boosting her immune system. As that system became stronger, the eczema also resolved.

A Case of Melasma

This phenomenon of everything falling into place when you treat the root problem applied to another patient, Mary. In her late forties, Mary came to see me for perimenopausal symptoms of frequent irregular bleeding and hot flashes. She also had an appointment with a dermatologist to treat the recent brownish discolorations on her face. She had a skin condition called melasma, felt to be caused by an imbalance in female hormones. Melasma is common during pregnancy and may or may not resolve after the pregnancy is over. The Western treatment for it is usually cosmetic, a topical bleaching agent. Once I treated Mary's menstrual irregularities with cycled doses of the hormone, progesterone, and then stabilized her hormonal balance with herbs, her melasma disappeared, and she no longer needed the bleaching agent.

Diabetic Nephropathy

My first patient, Betty, referred Wilma, who was thirty-three years old when she first came to see me. She had suffered from diabetes since the age of nine. The physician treating her diabetes had just told her that in a matter of five to six years she would need dialysis for kidney failure. At the time, 1985, other than monitoring kidney function, controlling the blood glucose, and perhaps prescribing a low protein diet, there were no known Western remedies to slow the progression of diabetic nephropathy. I treated Wilma using an herbal formula for glomerulonephritis that I had learned from Dr. Lai. The kidney is made of many units called glomeruli, which function as filters, allowing waste products to pass through their pores and into the urine without allowing the bigger molecules such as protein to be lost into the urine. In both glomerulonephritis and diabetic nephropathy, some of the kidney's glomeruli malfunction and allow protein to pass through into the urine. Wilma's prescription included herbs to tonify the Kidney, improving circulation to that area, Spleen herbs to help control her diabetes, and herbs often used for respiratory problems that protect the mucous membranes. The mucous membrane herbs help to normalize the filtering membrane of the glomeruli and not allow the pores to leak protein into the urine. By the time I retired from my integrated practice, Wilma, at age forty-nine, maintained her herbal regimen and still had not required dialysis.

Gallstones

Several years into my integrated practice, one of my Chinese church friends referred his sister to me. She was middle aged, slightly overweight, but otherwise in fair health. She described recurring symptoms of right upper abdominal pain that seemed to occur more when she ate fatty foods. My diagnosis of gallstones was confirmed by an ultrasound test. I recommended surgery, but she declined. Shortly thereafter, she returned home to Seattle. Time passed. One day I bumped into her in San Francisco, when she was again visiting her brother. She told me she had taken a patent Chinese herbal medicine called Dam Tong 膽通 (which means "opening up the gallbladder") and her gallstones had disappeared. This was confirmed by a repeat of her ultrasound in Seattle. Interesting, I thought, and filed the idea in the back of my mind.

Subsequently, Mrs. H., a Chinese Vietnamese refugee, came to see me with symptoms of gallstones. Her case was even more severe in that she had signs of liver dysfunction, indicating that the stones were obstructing the ducts that bring bile to the intestines. Again, the diagnosis was confirmed by ultrasound, and I recommended surgery. She asked if I knew of any other remedy. Understanding Chinese people's aversion to surgery, I told her my previous patient's story. I gave her the patent medicine name, Dam Tong, and told her she was on her own as far as trying to find the herbal medicine was concerned. I added that if it did not work, she should return promptly for surgery.

A few weeks later, she called to tell me she was having severe pain. I instructed her to go to the emergency room. A while after she arrived, the pain subsided. I strongly advised her to have surgery. She said, "I've been taking this herb medicine for about a month now. Why don't you order another ultrasound to see if my stones have disappeared?" I told her I believed the severe pain was an indication the stones were still present. Again, I urged her to have the surgery, and she finally agreed.

I arranged for her to have surgery by a Mandarin-speaking surgeon. Mrs. H. was quite anxious, having never set foot in a Western hospital before. Her son stayed with her to translate for her and give her moral support. The next day, the surgery was performed, and that evening I received a phone call from the surgeon. He removed the gallbladder, but to his surprise, there were no stones in it. He further commented that the operating field was quite bloody. (These were the pre-laparoscopic days, when gallbladders were removed under direct vision by opening up the abdomen.)

Later, at a Chinese Home Health facility where I taught a class, I encountered a physician from China. Immigrant physicians from China commonly encountered many obstacles to getting California medical licensure. They therefore often attended such classes in order to find work in a field related to medicine. I asked her if she knew about Dam Tong, and wondered if she knew how it worked to eliminate gallstones. She told me that the herbal formula acts by relaxing the smooth muscles, which is what makes up the walls of bile ducts and blood vessels. When the smooth muscles are relaxed, the ducts dilate, allowing stones, if small enough, to pass through into the intestines. As I reflected on Mrs. H.'s case, it made sense. The severe pain that had required emergency room admission was probably the stones passing from her bile duct into her intestines. When they finally passed, the pain subsided. When the surgeon operated, he found the operative field bloody because the blood vessels around the gallbladder area were also dilated from the Dam Tong.

After that incident, when any of my patients with gallstones requested an alternative to surgery, I gave them the option. If their condition fit the criteria for using ursodiol, a Western drug that can dissolve cholesterol gallstones, I prescribed it in conjunction with Dam Tong. I had found a source of the herb product in Hong Kong, but late in my practice, Dam Tong was no longer available there. Now, newer and equally effective herbal formulations can probably be found.

Peripheral Vascular Disease

Not long after I started my integrated practice, Ed referred one of his patients to me for hay fever and lower back pain. Mrs. A. was in her seventies. I treated her hay fever with herbs and used acupuncture for her back pain. Several months into her treatment course, Mrs. A. asked me if the acupuncture she was receiving also helped circulation. She told me that she had suffered from peripheral vascular disease, which was being monitored by a vascular surgeon. Before seeing me, she could walk only three blocks before leg pain would make her stop because the arteries to her legs were partially blocked. A few months after beginning TCM treatments, she noticed that she was able to walk at least twice as far without pain, and her vascular surgeon recently told her the Doppler examination of her legs showed improved blood flow.

I did not think acupuncture could be responsible for the improvement. Most likely it was the herbs. Shortly afterward, I attended a lecture on the results of research conducted in China on some commonly used Chinese herbs. The speaker told us herbs classified as "quelling Wind 驅風" (see chapter 4) improve circulation to the peripheral vascular system. Quelling Wind herbs were in Mrs. A.'s prescription for hay fever.

Since treating Mrs. A, I have used an herbal formula combining quelling Wind with mobilizing Qi and Blood 行氣活血 herbs (see chapter 3) for peripheral vascular occlusive disease. If the disease is not advanced, blood flow generally improves. I once treated an avid golfer who could play only nine holes without the use of a golf cart because of his claudication (calf pain caused by inadequate blood flow to the legs). After treatment, he was able to walk the entire eighteen holes. I have also treated diabetics with the typical nocturnal leg pain from peripheral vascular disease. One patient was in her eighties. On our initial respective examinations, neither her podiatrist nor I could feel the dorsalis pedis pulse in her foot. After my treatment, her pain disappeared, and the pulse became palpable.

Women's Health

Treating women's health problems with TCM has been one of the most gratifying aspects of my integrated practice. So often, women's complaints are written off by Western practitioners because they don't fit neatly into the Western diagnostic or therapeutic box. In the TCM paradigm, on the other hand, these symptoms not only make sense but are treatable.

Premenstrual Syndrome

One of my gynecology colleagues told me that when he was in training, what he most dreaded attending was the premenstrual syndrome (PMS) clinic, because there was so little that could be done for women suffering from PMS. But TCM shines in this area. I began treating women plagued with PMS, women who came in tearfully relating that they had only two good weeks out of each month. After I treated these women with herbs, their faces would light up with a smile on their return visits. For years, the prevailing Western medical belief was that PMS was only in the minds and emotions of women. Now, it is recognized that neurohumoral changes occur premenstrually. The current Western explanation is that PMS appears to come from an imbalance in the hormones secreted by the ovary. The current Western treatment of choice is antidepressant drugs, which have significant side effects (Grady-Weliky 2003). The Eastern approach is to use herbs that tonify Blood 補血, such as Angelica Sinensis 當歸, combined with herbs that improve circulation to the ovaries, such as Rhizoma Cyperi 香附. Using acupuncture to improve circulation to the ovaries is also effective. When the ovaries have an improved blood flow and are healthier, the hormone secretions become balanced, and the PMS symptoms resolve.

Menstrual Irregularities

Some women have irregular or infrequent periods because of a weak pituitary-ovarian axis. Normally, after puberty, the pituitary gland secretes FSH, a hormone that stimulates ovulation. When ovulation occurs, the egg releases estrogen and progesterone into the blood, and the pituitary gland shuts off and does not stimulate the ovaries again until the egg, if not fertilized, dies. The blood levels of the two hormones fall when the unfertilized egg dies, menstruation ensues, and a new cycle begins again with the pituitary secreting FSH.

Western practitioners treat irregular periods with birth control pills, which contain estrogen and progesterone, fooling the pituitary gland to go into its shut-off mode. During the last seven days of the birth control pill cycle, no hormones are taken, the blood levels of estrogen and progesterone fall, and the result is an artificially induced period. After the seven days, the woman resumes taking the hormones. Sensing the hormones, the pituitary gland continues to shut off FSH production, and the ovaries remain unstimulated. If the pill is taken for years, the unstimulated ovaries can "forget" to ovulate. The regular periods induced by birth control pills, like window dressing, make for a good Biao 表, but there is absolutely no benefit for the Ben 本.

For the purpose of contraception, the pill makes sense. For normalizing a weak system in women interested in eventual fertility, it is counterproductive. Herbs and acupuncture, on the other hand, can increase blood flow to the reproductive system and encourage ovarian function to normalize. Allopathic physicians, unaware of this complementary approach, prescribe the pill because for them, there are no other options.

Colds and Flus

One winter day during the flu season, Ed told me he had to take home some sample medication to his wife who was ill with the flu. He asked me to suggest an antibiotic. I told him, "You know the flu is caused by a virus, and antibiotics have no known effect on viruses." "I know," he said, "but I have to bring her something. She's my wife." Using antibiotics to treat the flu is one example of how allopathic physicians sometimes treat for the sake of fulfilling patient expectations, whether rational or not.

The allopathic medical community acknowledges that the most common overuse of antibiotics is for bronchitis. This overuse has led to an alarming problem: the emergence of strains of bacteria resistant to existing antibiotics. Pharmaceutical companies are constantly doing research to design newer drugs to outsmart the resistant bacteria. In order to recoup research expenses and make a profit, they market the new drugs extensively. Part of the marketing strategy is to give plenty of samples to physicians who, when faced with social pressures such as in Ed's case, perpetuate this overuse. In many instances, a complementary approach is far less harmful. Some Chinese herbs are known to have antiviral properties. I have often found using these herbs, along with immune-boosting herbs, an effective way to treat colds and flu early and prevent bronchitis from developing.

Hyperactive Airway Disease

I realized I had come full circle in my integrated practice when my mother's friend enlisted my help for her post-flu cough, a dry, hacking cough that her son, the chest specialist, could not cure. That type of cough was exactly what I had as a third-year medical student when my mother took me to the herbalist. I dutifully used TCM methods to examine her, remembering Dr. Lai's words: "Any TCM doctor is not worth his salt if he can't treat a dry, hacking cough. You just tonify the lung Yin." I prescribed the herbs, and after a week, her cough was gone.

Four years into my integrated practice, I outgrew my timeshare office and moved into my own space. When I first opened my practice, I received gifts of plants from friends and well-wishers. Perhaps because of overwatering, none survived under my brown thumb except for one, a Creeping Charlie plant. As I packed to move, I congratulated my Creeping Charlie, telling it, "You are my only surviving plant that I took care of regularly for four years." I picked up the pot and found it was very light. Evidently, my survivor was plastic! It survived not because of my care but in spite of it. I tell this story because we as healers often attribute success to our own efforts when actually it comes from the durable nature of the human body. TCM recognizes the body's innate healing power and employs treatments that enhance that power.

Chapter 9
Advanced TCM

During the early years of my integrated practice, I continued to study at Dr. Lai's once a week. The pragmatist in me used TCM formulas and was gratified by good results, but the scientist in me still wanted to know more. What did TCM teachings actually mean? How and why did they work? As my knowledge increased, I was able to connect the dots.

More about TCM Organs

Discovering that TCM organs were not the same as the organs Westerners knew by the same names left me in a quandary. Since the TCM terms Liver, Spleen, and Kidney actually meant entire physiologic systems, what terms do TCM practitioners use when they want to refer to the actual organs?

Liver 肝

If the TCM Liver represents the adrenergic and sympathetic nervous system, then how does TCM address problems with the actual organ that Westerners know as the liver? Actually, in ancient times,

TCM did not really know the organ as we understand it today. In antiquity, if someone had hepatitis, it was called Yellow Gallbladder 黃膽. Similarly, the Western lay term for hepatitis was yellow jaundice. These terms were descriptive. The skin and the whites of the eyes turn yellow in hepatitis patients because their livers' ability to process and eliminate pigment from the breakdown of red blood cells is impaired. The TCM treatment for this condition is to clear Heat and cleanse toxins. Since hepatitis is usually from a viral infection, this treatment is appropriate. Today, the cause of Yellow Gallbladder is known, and there is a Chinese term for hepatitis, liver inflammation 肝 炎. The treatment principle of clearing Heat and cleansing toxin remains the same.

The TCM practitioner would diagnose cirrhosis, another disease of the liver, as hardening of the liver 肝 硬 化. The TCM treatment is directed at improving circulation to the liver and dispersing scar tissue. When the TCM practitioner diagnoses Liver Fire 肝火 or Liver Yang rising up 肝火上升, however, he is talking about an overactive sympathetic nervous system, and he then uses calming Liver Fire 調和肝火 herbs, which decrease sympathetic activity. Therefore, it appears that when we hear the term "liver," in order to know what the TCM practitioner is referring to, we have to consider the context.

Kidney 腎

I had the same question about the kidney. If the TCM Kidney represents the reproductive system, what about treatment for diseases of the actual kidney? As it does with the liver, TCM treats diseases of the kidney with appropriate herbal formulas. If there is a kidney infection, the TCM principle is to clear heat and cleanse toxins with a group of herbs that are effective against the commonly known bacteria involved in kidney infections. If a patient's kidney is failing, the TCM practitioner says that the patient's kidney function is low. With common signs of aging, the TCM practitioner says the Kidney is deficient. Again, context is the key.

Kidney 腎 and Life Gate 命門

Although the concept of Life Gate was presented in early lessons at my TCM school, I neither understood it nor paid much attention to it. It sounded like just another metaphor for life and death. As my understanding increased, I ventured into analyzing this concept further.

At ACTCM, the lecturer had said:

> *"Life Gate is closely related to kidney Qi. Life Gate is the fountainhead of Yuan or Original Qi; it is the root of all organs and root of all meridians; it is the door of breathing, the springhead of Triple Burner Qi; it is the abode of original Yang, compared to the kidney, which is the abode of original Yin. Original Yang is congenital fire. Original Yin is congenital water. Water and fire, Yin and Yang must be in equilibrium. If the Qi of Life Gate dies, life ends."*

Dr. Lai also used to say, "Death comes when the life gate closes."

The epiphany came one day. What happens when someone dies? The heart stops. What do we do when we witness the heart stopping? We start CPR and then reach for adrenaline to try to restart the heart. One part of the adrenal gland, the medulla, makes adrenaline and noradrenaline. Both stimulate the heart to beat stronger. Noradrenaline constricts blood vessels to increase blood pressure, while Adrenaline makes the heart beat faster and stronger. The adrenal gland is always stimulated whenever there is a crisis, whether physical or emotional. I concluded that at least part of the Life Gate concept includes the adrenal medulla, which represents both *fire* 火 and *original Yang* 原陽氣.

The other part of the adrenal gland, the cortex, makes steroids, which tone down inflammation, a Yin function. Besides cortisol, this part of the adrenal gland also makes aldosterone, a hormone that helps the body retain fluid, also a Yin function. In this context, if Life Gate is the adrenal medulla, at least part of the TCM Kidney is the adrenal cortex. It is *water,* or *original Yin,* 原 陰 氣. The teaching that *"Water and fire, Yin and Yang must be in equilibrium"* makes Western sense when all aspects of the adrenal gland are taken into consideration.

The TCM Kidney is far more complex than I had earlier conceived it to be. It encompasses not only the reproductive system but also the adrenal cortex and, as mentioned earlier, the bone marrow (see chapter 2). The bone marrow produces red and white blood cells, among which are B-lymphocytes, responsible for antibody production. The immune system, then, must be included in the Kidney concept as well.

Spleen 脾

My feeling about the TCM Spleen can best be expressed with the words Winston Churchill used to describe Russia's war strategy during WWII: "It is a riddle wrapped in a mystery inside an enigma." With the passage of time and new discoveries in Western medicine, I have been able to unwrap some layers of the enigma surrounding the riddle of the TCM Spleen. From my early days studying TCM, I knew that the Spleen concept included the digestive system and water metabolism. Yet the way Dr. Lai used Spleen herbs made me think it had to involve more. He used them to boost the immune system and to treat obesity. He told me people with Spleen deficiency 脾虛 have a craving for sweets. When the Spleen is tonified, the craving goes away and they lose weight. He often pointed out the typical physical sign of a pale swollen tongue in patients with Spleen deficiency. What did all these swollen tongues signify? The things he taught about treating the Spleen prompted me to review my ACTCM class notes:

> *The spleen governs transporting nutrition: absorption and digestion of food. Every part of the body depends on the spleen meridian for nutrition. After birth, the spleen is essential. It nurtures body Yin and earth. Its nature is damp, but it dislikes dampness. Spleen Qi*

must be rising to be normal. Only if spleen Qi is rising
does nutrition derived from food go all over. If spleen
Qi is deficient, symptoms are anorexia, edema, and
diarrhea; dampness is congested in the body.

The Spleen and Glucose Metabolism

Mary was a rather plump woman who attended occasional classes at ACTCM. After I left the school, I happened to ask Dr. Lai about her. He told me she was no longer overweight because he had treated her Spleen. Putting together what Dr. Lai taught about Spleen-deficient patients craving sweets and the success in treating Mary's obesity with Spleen-tonifying herbs, I reasoned that the TCM Spleen must have something to do with glucose metabolism.

Normally, the food we eat is absorbed and changed to glucose that is carried in the blood. Glucose needs to enter muscle cells to provide them with energy. To understand the action of insulin, it helps to imagine that the muscle cell has a door with a lock. Insulin unlocks the door to let the glucose into the muscle cell. After the muscles take up the needed amount of glucose from the blood, the excess glucose is stored in the liver as glycogen. Whenever the muscles need more glucose, such as during exercise, the liver changes the glycogen back into glucose and releases it into the blood to again supply the muscle cells.

In type 2 diabetes, the body makes insulin, but the muscle cell lock changes, making it more difficult for insulin to open the door and let in glucose. This is called insulin resistance. The result is excess glucose levels in the blood. Adding to the problem is that the liver in type 2 diabetes seems to release too much glucose into the blood. The body reacts by making more and more insulin trying to overcome the problem. Excess insulin causes a multitude of maladies, among which are hypertension and obesity.

First-generation diabetes drugs stimulate the pancreas to produce more insulin. Second-generation diabetes drugs act in one of two ways. One class, the thiazolidinediones (TZDs), helps glucose get into muscle cells more easily. The undesirable side effect is that with improved insulin sensitivity, patients gain weight on TZDs. Another downside risk under investigation is a possible increase in cardiovascular complications among users of the TZD, Rosiglitazone (Nissen and Wolski 2007). The other class of second-generation drugs prevents the liver from releasing too much glucose. Metformin falls into this second category. Metformin encourages weight loss but it cannot be prescribed in patients with poor kidney function, and there is a danger of lactic acidosis when taken by extremely ill patients. Studies have shown that the Spleen herb, Radix Astragali 黃其 improves the liver's ability to keep glucose stored as glycogen, similar to the action of metformin. Another Spleen herb, Atractyloidis Alba 白朮 is known to lower blood sugar, but the mechanism has not been clarified.

A recent breakthrough discovery is that the intestines secrete a group of hormones called incretins, which act in several ways to counter the progression of type 2 diabetes (Ratner 2005). Incretins decrease the liver's output of glucose, improve the efficiency of the pancreas by stimulating it to produce insulin only when the blood glucose is high, make food stay in the stomach longer so that the person feels full and eats less, and enhances the longevity of pancreatic beta cells responsible for making insulin. Since the TCM Spleen concept includes the digestive system, tonifying the system should help diabetics by enhancing incretin secretion. A drug is now available for enhancing incretin levels, but it needs to be injected.

Obesity leading to type 2 diabetes mellitus has reached epidemic proportions in developed countries. While the solution lies mainly in lifetsyle modification—changing eating habits and increasing exercise—using TCM treatments that tonify the Spleen can be an important adjunct.

The Spleen and the Immune System

Another enigmatic Spleen concept has been the meaning of "*Its nature is damp, but it dislikes dampness.*" When Dr. Lai treated patients with Spleen deficiency, patients who exhibited the typical pale, swollen tongues, he often said, "The problem here is wetness, causing congestion. We need to clean the Wet and clear it." It is common for TCM terminology such as "clean the Wet 去濕" to sound incomplete to a Westerner. Clean the Wet from what? I had to remember that without a microscope or the knowledge of anatomy, that was as far as TCM could go with explanations. When I asked Dr. Lai why Spleen-deficient patients seemed to show these signs of water retention, he said it was from inflammation. I asked how that led to water retention. He said it was because of capillary leakage. His answer reminded me of what I learned about Wetness when I studied the Six Evils (see chapter 4).

Western medicine now recognizes that inflammation gives rise to a multitude of diseases such as clogged arteries and cancer. Inflammation is a nonspecific response by the immune system. With inflammation, the body attacks foreign invaders and becomes a war zone with dead white blood cells, dead foreign cells, and the fluid from capillary leakage. Normally, the immune system has T-Helper cells that direct fighting cells where to go and what to attack when there is an invader. The same immune system also has T-Suppressor cells that direct fighting cells when it is time to quit. Macrophages, also part of the immune system, eat up debris, and the lymphatic system carries the debris and excess fluid away from tissue and back into the circulation. In Spleen-deficient patients, the inflammatory response is inappropriate and prolonged. Fluid and debris in tissues may accumulate at a rate greater than the capacity of the cleanup mechanisms to remove them.

The TCM Spleen includes the thymus and lymphoid tissue, which produce the T-cell component of the immune system. It also includes the lymphatic system, which carries away debris and excess fluid. *Its nature is damp* means that the Spleen tends to generate an immune response, which involves capillary leakage. *It dislikes dampness* describes the normal function the immune system has of cleaning up after itself. Spleen-tonifying herbs help to normalize the immune system. They enhance not only the inflammatory phase but also the cease and desist and cleanup phase of immune function. The Spleen herb Radix Astragali 黃耆 boosts immunity by stimulating T cell production. Other Spleen herbs such as Radix Diascoreae Oppositae 山藥 and Atractylodis Alba 白朮 have diuretic properties. They enhance macrophage function and facilitate fluid mobilization by the lymphatics.

Further revisiting the Spleen, I analyzed its other descriptions.

The spleen governs blood. It controls and regulates the direction of blood. If it malfunctions, the symptom is a deficient type of bleeding. The *deficient type of bleeding* is described here in contrast to bleeding from Heat conditions. In Heat conditions, there is inflammation. Blood tends to rush to inflamed areas where dilated blood vessels, when broken, will bleed profusely, such as in cases of tuberculosis or dysentery. Deficient bleeding, on the other hand, occurs in conditions where the patient is debilitated and does not suffer from a Heat condition or infection. I pondered for a long time over the meaning of the term *regulates the direction of blood*. To my Western mind, it is the heart's pumping action that determines the direction of the blood. If blood is not pumped forward, the only other direction is backward, and that leads to heart failure, not bleeding. As I read more about the TCM theory of bleeding, it occurred to me that the ancients viewed bleeding as a problem of blood traveling in the wrong direction. A flashback came: The ancients were not aware of the cardiovascular system nor was the clotting mechanism clear to them. The cause of *deficient type of bleeding* is actually an abnormality in part of the clotting mechanism. Protein is needed for the bone marrow to make clotting factors. Absorption of protein depends on a normal digestive system, and digestion is part of the Spleen's function.

The spleen governs muscle, goes all the way to the mouth, and flourishes in the lips. If his spleen is strong, the person is muscular and lips are red. Strong muscles and healthy lip color are signs of good nutrition, all of which TCM attributes to a healthy Spleen that actually represents the digestive system.

If spleen Qi is deficient, there is anorexia, edema, and diarrhea, meaning dampness is congested in the body. If we consider the Spleen as the digestive system, poor function leading to malabsorption can explain these symptoms. If we consider the TCM Spleen as representing the immune system, there is yet another explanation for the symptom of diarrhea. Diarrhea was a hallmark symptom of HIV-AIDS during the early days of the epidemic when the HIV virus had not yet been discovered. Later, we learned that these patients commonly suffered from intestinal infections that their immune systems were too weak to overcome. A weak immune system can lead to infectious diarrhea.

TCM Organ Interrelationships

The idea of one organ attacking or sustaining another organ, as taught in TCM, confounded my Western-trained mind. For a long time I simply discarded the dogma because I couldn't make sense of it. It was not until much later that I understood what these inter-relationships meant. I realized that the organs they talked about were not really organs but physiologic systems that interacted with one another.

Liver 肝 and Spleen 脾

For years, I puzzled over the TCM teaching: *If liver Qi is congested, it invades the spleen. Symptoms are anorexia, diarrhea, and poor digestion.* I kept questioning how one organ could invade another. One day the answer came to me. The TCM Liver is the sympathetic nervous system, which is turned on with stress. The opposing system is the parasympathetic, normally turned on for nonstressful states like digestion. One of the Spleen's functions is digestion. It is obvious that when we are stressed, our digestion suffers. Sometimes we lose our appetites, and after a meal, we feel gaseous. That is because the overactive sympathetic system has overridden the parasympathetic system. The Liver has invaded the Spleen. I was in awe of how much sense this made.

Kidney 腎 and Lung 肺

More than one teacher at ACTCM taught us that in order to treat the Lung, we must also treat the Kidney. I used to follow this dictum when writing my herb prescriptions, not fully understanding the reasoning behind it. When I came to understand that the Kidney represented the adrenal cortex, which makes steroids, the connection with the lung became clearer. In recent years, Western practitioners recognize that inflammation plays a major role in asthma, and they recommend using steroid inhalers for asthma. If the TCM Kidney is the steroid-producing part of the adrenal gland, it makes perfect sense to enhance the Kidney to treat inflammatory lung conditions. It also makes sense when we consider the Kidney's role in antibody formation as a producer of marrow. Most respiratory infections require efficient antibody formation to control the infectious invader, be it bacterial, viral, or fungal. A Western-trained physician might then question whether Kidney herbs are comparable to synthetic estrogens or steroids. Kidney herbs do not have the known side effects of synthetic hormones. They most likely act by improving blood flow to various glands.

Liver 肝, Spleen 脾, Kidney 腎, and Lung 肺

Dr. Lai often said, "For lung diseases, we have to calm the Liver 調和肝 to stop it from attacking the Spleen, as well as support the Spleen and Kidney 健脾補腎 to treat the Lung 養肺." It was only when I used the TCM meaning of these various organs that I could understand his algorithm.

When we are emotionally stressed, our sympathetic system, the TCM Liver, is overactive. This overactive Liver, or sympathetic system, suppresses our normal digestion and immune response, represented by the TCM Spleen. Thus, the Liver needs to be calmed in order to allow proper Spleen function. The TCM Spleen includes the immune system, which is needed to ward off infection; therefore, we need to "support the Spleen." Finally, the TCM Kidney, responsible for steroid production and antibody formation, should be tonified to control inflammation and boost immunity.

When I found this rather whimsical ancient depiction of human anatomy (fig. 6), I realized that six hollow organs (regarded mostly as conduits) and five solid organs plus the Life Gate were all the ancients knew about to explain diverse biological phenomena. It is understandable that they assigned functions of various organs, such as glands that they did not know about to their limited organ repertoire. The assignments may lack the precision familiar to Westerners. Spleen and Stomach are often used together, especially when diagnosing deficiencies. Kidney and Life Gate are frequently mentioned in tandem. Various brain functions were designated to several different organs. The cerebral cortex went to the Heart and Kidney. The amygdala, the area responsible for rage, went to the Liver. The adrenal medulla was assigned to the Liver and Life Gate. Of additional interest is the written explanation

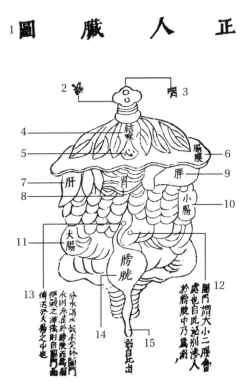

Fig. 6. Ancient Anatomical Diagram of Human Organs, courtesy of the *Bibliotheque Nationale de France, Paris* (Lyons and Petrucelli 1987, 126).

1. Normal Human Organ Anatomy; 2. Hypopharynx; 3. Pharynx; 4. Thyroid Cartilage; 5. Heart; 6. Diaphragm; 7. Liver; 8. Stomach; 9. Spleen; 10. Small Intestines; 11. Large Intestines; 12. Dividing Gate is the junction of small and large intestines; 13. At Dividing Gate, the remains of ingested food, after absorption and digestion, are separated into clear liquid, which is excreted through the bladder as urine, and solid, which is excreted through the colon as feces; 14. Bladder; 15. Urine is excreted here.

of how urine is made—at the junction of the small and large intestine where they thought solid and liquid waste are separated. The ancients did not realize that the kidney is the organ that makes urine. It is amazing nevertheless that the ancient Chinese, despite their limited knowledge of anatomy, were able to devise a workable system of diagnosis and develop some very effective, appropriate, and enduring treatments. Table 4 depicts TCM organ assignments.

Table 4. TCM Organ Assignments

HEART	LUNG	LIVER	SPLEEN/STOMACH	KIDNEY	LIFE GATE
Brain	Lung	Sympathetic N.S. Adrenal Medulla Brain	Stomach Small Intestines Pancreas Thymus Lymphatic System Parasympathetic N.S.	Testes Ovaries Bone Marrow Adrenal Cortex Brain	Adrenal Medulla

Modern Applications of the Eight Entities 八大綱

I found that most of TCM teaching was about infectious diseases. With modern antibiotics and vaccination programs, treating infectious diseases with TCM seemed obsolete. Today, the Western focus is on degenerative diseases and cancer. I sought to find how this ancient system could be adapted to contemporary needs.

Heat 熱 and Solid 實 Conditions

Viral infections represent a frontier the West has not completely conquered. People are still getting sick with colds and flus. Recent challenges include SARS, the West Nile virus, and Avian flu. We have been far more successful at developing antibiotics to treat bacterial infections because bacteria are complete living cells, making them easier to analyze. We can actually grow them in a lab, study their biology, and design drugs to kill them by foiling some stage of their multiplication and growth. Viruses, on the other hand, are incomplete cells. They need to parasitize a host cell and borrow its cell biology in order to grow and multiply, making them more difficult to study. Western drugs are designed with specificity. If we cannot analyze a virus or understand its metabolism, we cannot design our bullet to target it. The most effective Western approach for fighting viruses is to develop vaccines, but vaccine development takes time and requires intimate knowledge of how the virus acts. We are constantly threatened by new and unfamiliar viruses because there will always be a lag between when diseases occur and when vaccines are available.

TCM offers a nonspecific approach to treating viral infections. TCM practitioners do not have to pinpoint the exact infecting agent to treat. Viruses are classified as Heat toxins, against which the host mounts a Solid or immune response. I once asked Dr. Lai, "How can you know that the cleansing toxins and clearing Heat herbs you use for flu can kill the virus when the specific flu virus hasn't been identified?" He told me that these herbs may not be working on just the one level to kill viruses but may also down-regulate the host's Solid response to the infection, such as high fever and severe lung inflammation. Often what causes death with severe infections is not the invader but the patient's own extreme response to infection. With severe pneumonia, for instance, the lung tissue gets so inflamed that oxygen cannot pass through the swollen air sacs of the lung to get to the blood. With the SARS epidemic, it was after the virus was no longer detectable that severe respiratory failure set in, and steroids were used in an attempt to diminish the inflammatory reaction. TCM clearing-Heat herbs may similarly decrease the inflammation without the side effects of steroids. Combinations of these herbs are quite effective for colds, the flu, and viral gastroenteritis (stomach flu). In fact, some common formulas of these herbs are available in either pill form or other forms such as powder or bouillon cubes easily reconstituted with hot water. They are sold over the counter in herbal shops or even in Chinese supermarkets. For colds and flus, preparations of Yin-qiao 銀翹, Ban Lan Gen 板藍根, or Gum Wall 金和 tea are available; for viral gastroenteritis, Huang Lien Shang Ching Pien 黃連上清片 is.

Despite advances in antimicrobial and antiparasitic development, we face the constant challenge of drug resistance. It seems that bacteria and parasites, by the process of mutation and natural selection, are constantly developing new strains that are resistant to existing drugs. This problem is worsened by physicians' overprescribing antibiotics and by the drug companies' development of longer-acting antibiotics, which are very popular because of their convenience. Some antibiotics need to be taken only once instead of the usual ten days. Evidently, the long-acting nature of new antibiotics allows the active ingredient in the blood to become lowered to the point that some hardy bacteria survive the treatment to return with a vengeance another day. In many parts of the world, drug-resistant malaria is becoming prevalent, and the World Health Organization is recommending treatment with the herb Artimesia Apiaceae 青蒿 (Vega and Barclay 2005, 1–5). The herb Pulsatillae Chinensis 白頭翁 is known to be effective for amoebic dysentery. Other herbs in the cold-cleansing category have been shown to have antibacterial activity and warrant further studies. Resorting to herbal remedies may become an option for other infections where drug resistance is a problem.

We are just beginning to find out that many conditions, such as arteriosclerosis and tumors, which in the past were considered degenerative, actually start from an inflammatory process. Some cancers, and even heart disease, are linked to infections. Cervical cancer is caused by human papillomavirus. As for heart disease, there is possible association between it and certain infections (Wierzbicki and Hagmeyer 2000). Heart disease and tumors are not mentioned much in ancient TCM literature because people commonly died of infectious diseases and simply did not live long enough to acquire these other ailments. With current knowledge, we can categorize these conditions as Heat and Solid. Herbs for clearing Heat 清熱 and cleansing toxins 解毒 have potential use in these cases.

Deficiency 虛 Conditions

The Deficient 虛 state occurred in antiquity often as the aftermath of a severe infection when the patient became weak and exhausted. Today, while people do not so commonly suffer from the ravages of severe infection, the Deficiency state still exists, but the cause has changed: now the Deficient state is from the stress of modern life. This was true in most of my patients. Thus, various TCM tonifying herbs to restore energy are still relevant to today's patients.

Blood Stasis and Ecchymosis 血瘀

Cardiovascular diseases constitute the leading cause of death in Western countries and continue to be the focus of intense research into prevention as well as treatment. Any discussion of modern application of TCM would be incomplete without mentioning the treatment of Blood Stasis and Ecchymosis as it applies to cardio-vascular disease. The term, vitalizing or mobilizing blood 活血, used to puzzle me. Blood has no ability to move of its own accord; it moves because the heart and blood vessels control it. In order to make sense of this term, I needed to remind myself that the ancients had an incomplete knowledge of the cardiovascular system, which they called Qi. Often in TCM, "moving blood" 活血 and "moving Qi" 行氣 are used together. Herbs in this category move Qi by dilating blood vessels to improve circulation. They move blood (also known as dispersing blood 散血) by thinning it, somewhat like aspirin. If the blood is thinner and the blood vessels are dilated, it will "move" better. Moving-blood and moving-Qi herbs are comparable to vaso-dilators and antiplatelet drugs commonly used for coronary heart disease that dilate blood vessels and thin blood. The West could benefit from further investigating these herbs and considering them as either potential adjuncts to Western therapy or alternatives when patients do not tolerate drugs such as aspirin.

With time and patience, I slowly found answers to many of my questions. In my TCM journey, I learned to persevere and constantly keep in mind the meanings behind its unique terminology.

Chapter 10

About Acupuncture

While the Western medical establishment continues to ruminate over whether this ancient therapy has validity, patients who have been treated successfully with acupuncture are convinced of its effectiveness. Demand for acupuncture is growing, not waning. Its safety record trumps that of drugs and epidural steroids. Although it cannot fit neatly into the box Western science has set up as the only acceptable gold standard—randomized, double blind, placebo-controlled study—neither can surgery. Let us explore what is known about it.

Frequently Asked Questions about Acupuncture

What are acupuncture channels or meridians 經脈?

I have puzzled over what acupuncture channels or meridians are for years. Do they represent the vascular system? While most channels run vertically throughout the body like the circulatory system, their course and interconnections are not the same as the circulatory system. Do channels represent the nervous system? While acupuncture points 穴位 often fall along some part of peripheral nerves, their channel pathways do not correspond to nervous system pathways. How each channel is connected to a specific organ has also baffled me. For instance, why do we use a point along the Large Intestine channel located on the hand to treat facial pain?

A review of the history of acupuncture might shed some light. Acupuncture was discovered by serendipity. In ancient times, the Chinese found that sometimes when they accidentally struck or injured a certain point on the body, it seemed to relieve certain conditions. I can imagine how a warrior, having been struck by a spear or arrow to his back, might have awakened the next morning and realized that his nagging back pain had disappeared.

With some conditions, they found that pressing on certain locations on the body caused pain. These locations were called ashi 阿是 points. "Ashi" literally means "ah, yes," an exclamation I often hear when I examine patients and press on a sore spot, which I would then acupuncture. When these points were stimulated by either pressure or massage, punctured with animal bones, or warmed with heat by holding burning mugwort leaf 艾葉 near them, the condition seemed to improve. Stimulating a certain point on the lower leg (St 36), for instance, relieved stomachaches. Pressure on a point on the hand (LI 4) relieved toothaches. Some of these points, we now know, correspond to Western trigger points. Other points are known to conduct electricity better than their surrounding tissue, and anatomically they often coincide with points on peripheral nerves; still others coincide with nerve roots as they come out of the spine. The observation that stimulating certain locations on the body surface had a therapeutic effect on certain conditions was first recorded in 300 BC in the *Inner Classic* 內 經 (a compilation of medical teachings transmitted orally as early as 2674 BC and put into writing in 300 BC). The ancients deduced that somehow these reactive points on the body surface are connected to remote parts of the body and to internal organs through pathways. With only a rudimentary knowledge of anatomy, TCM healers devised their system of mapping these pathways and called them channels or meridians. It is as if someone, looking at the doors and windows on the outside of a house, mapped its floor plan.

The primary channels number one to twelve. Each bears the name of the organ to which it is connected. Pathways along the back were named after the six fu (hollow) organs, and are classified as Yang. Those in the front of the body are named after zhang (solid) organs, and are classified as Yin. There are only five zhang organs, but that did not pose an insurmountable problem for the Chinese. Just as they added an extra season to fit the Five Phases theory (see chapter 4), they simply added one more organ, the Pericardium, so that the primary Yin channels also totaled six. Later, two more channels, the Conception channel, traversing the front midline of the body, and the Governing channel, traversing the back midline, were added. Some points not on the original twelve channels were later found to have therapeutic effects on internal organs. Additional channels were then mapped, and these were called the Miscellaneous channels, Divergent channels, Connecting channels, and Muscle channels. With time, more points with therapeutic effects were found, and these were called Extraordinary Points.

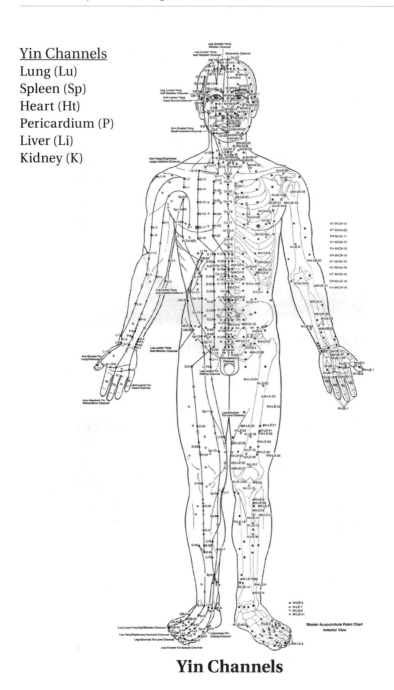

Yin Channels

Lung (Lu)
Spleen (Sp)
Heart (Ht)
Pericardium (P)
Liver (Li)
Kidney (K)

Yin Channels

Fig. 7a. Yin Acupuncture Channels.

Reprinted with permission of Redwing Press (O'Connor 1981 centerfold)

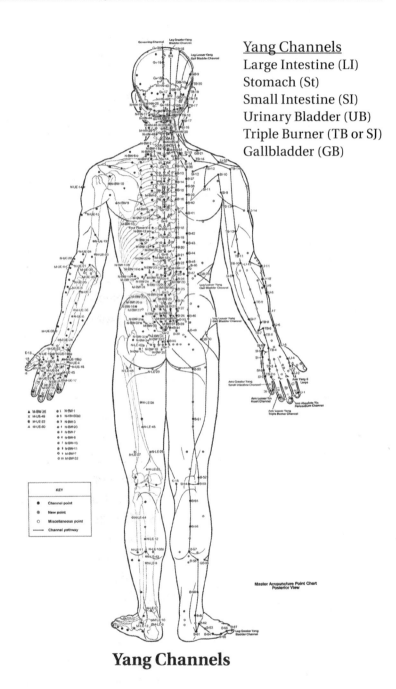

Yang Channels
Large Intestine (LI)
Stomach (St)
Small Intestine (SI)
Urinary Bladder (UB)
Triple Burner (TB or SJ)
Gallbladder (GB)

Yang Channels

Fig. 7b. Yang Acupuncture Channels.
Reprinted with permission of Redwing Press (O'Connor 1981 centerfold)

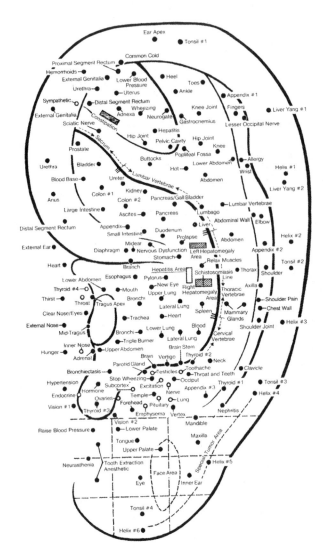

Fig. 8. Ear Acupuncture Points.
Reprinted with the permission of Eastland Press (O'Connor and Bensky 1981, 478).

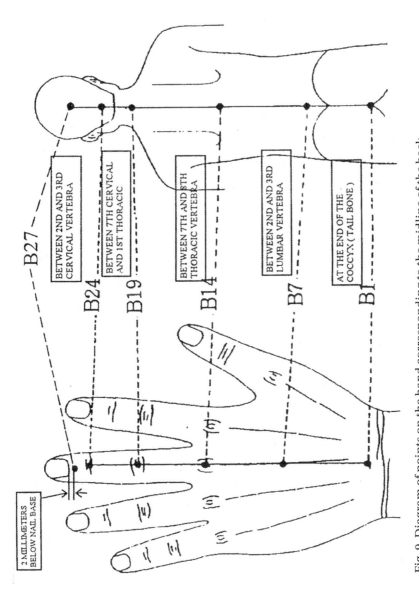

2 MILLIMETERS BELOW NAIL BASE

B27 —

BETWEEN 2ND AND 3RD CERVICAL VERTEBRA

B24

BETWEEN 7TH CERVICAL AND 1ST THORACIC

B19

BETWEEN 7TH AND 8TH THORACIC VERTEBRA

B14

BETWEEN 2ND AND 3RD LUMBAR VERTEBRA

B7

AT THE END OF THE COCCYX (TAIL BONE)

B1

Fig. 9. Diagram of points on the hand corresponding to the midline of the back.

Koryo Hand Therapy, 1997. Reprinted with the permission of Dan Lobash, Ph.D., L.Ac., Hemet, California.

The Western way of naming acupuncture points by their sequential number along channels is rather dull and unimaginative when compared to the Chinese names, which are descriptive and paint a word picture of the points. The acupuncture point below the lateral malleolus (the outer anklebone), named Kunlun, is one I frequently used when treating lumbosacral disc disease with pain radiation to the leg. Kunlun is the name of the mountain range separating Xinjiang Province from Tibet. When they looked at the protuberant anklebone, the Chinese saw a mountain. Anyone would agree that the name Kunlun is far more interesting than "Urinary Bladder 60."

Do these points on the skin actually connect to the internal organs along a pathway called a channel? It is difficult to determine. We need to keep in mind that some TCM organs represent physiologic systems rather than actual organs. An acupuncture chart will show channels traveling to organs like the liver, kidney, and spleen. Are the channel maps actually depicting an anatomical pathway leading to various organs, or are they just showing that the acupuncture points influence the physiologic systems that these organs represent? My best estimation is that some channel pathways, such as the Conception Channel that travels to the reproductive organs, are anatomical, while others are like diagrams pointing to what physiologic systems are affected by the acupuncture points on the channel. Shen Men 神門 (Heart 7), for instance, a point on the Heart Channel situated on the ulnar nerve at the wrist, is commonly used for sedation. The Chinese translation of Shen Men is "spirit door." The TCM Heart actually represents the nervous system. Points on the Heart Channel are not necessarily for treating cardiac problems.

What is even more confounding is that acupuncture points used to treat diseases pertaining to an organ are not necessarily located on that organ channel. To treat constipation, logic would guide you to find points on the Large Intestine channel. Actually, the best points for constipation are found on the Stomach channel. The best point for treating nausea, instead of being on the Stomach channel, is on the Pericardium channel. For treating urinary bladder problems, the best points are not found on the Urinary Bladder channel but on the Stomach and Conception channels. I have concluded that it is more expedient to learn which acupuncture points benefit which condition than to try to select points on the basis of channels alone.

What are the various types of acupuncture?

Body acupuncture was established during the third century BC. Since then, acupuncture microsystems have been discovered. These microsystems are representations (somewhat like maps) of the entire body on various body parts such as the ear, the hand, and the scalp. Acupuncturing the appropriate points on these body parts can also have therapeutic effects. Of these, I have used ear and hand acupuncture.

Ear Acupuncture: Chinese medical literature mentioned needling the ear to treat diseases as early as the Tang dynasty (AD 618–906). But it was a French physician named Nogier who expanded on this concept and developed a comprehensive system of ear acupuncture in the 1950s. A map of the entire body can be found on the ear. This map is laid out like an inverted fetus. In general, points for the head are located around the ear lobe; those for the feet, at the top of the ear. The Chinese used a standard map (see fig. 8), but the French have taken this to a higher level. They opine that the map can vary for different individuals, and they use intricate methods to determine which map a particular person has. The average acupuncturist, however, either by using a standard ear map and an electrical point detector, or by observing the location of skin changes on the ear, can determine which points to needle. I was amazed that I could see actual dryness and peeling of the skin over an Ear point representing a diseased area in the body. Asthmatics, for instance, often have skin changes over the Lung point. Some acupuncturists use ear acupuncture exclusively. I often combined ear acupuncture with body acupuncture for synergy.

For addictive behavior, acupuncture can be effective in relieving withdrawal symptoms but does not alter behavior. There is a Hunger point on the ear, but obese patients rarely overeat because of hunger. So I tell patients that acupuncture will not make them change their lifestyles but can help them maintain new ones when they have decided to change. I used to insert an indwelling needle on the Ear Shen Men point to help alleviate withdrawal symptoms when patients decided to stop smoking, but I worried about potential infections. Later, I taped small beads on that point. Much later, I showed the patients where the point was and taught them to pinch it themselves when they had a craving for a cigarette. One patient, for whom I prescribed the nicotine patch as well as this technique, was so afraid of the side effects of the patch when she read the package insert that she decided to just pinch her ears, and was able to stop smoking.

Korean Hand Acupuncture: Korean hand acupuncture is another twentieth century development. Like so many other advances in medicine, it was discovered by serendipity. The founder of this technique, Dr. Tae-Woo Yoo, wrote that one Autumn night in 1971, he was awakened from sleep by a pain in the back of his head so severe that he could not sleep. Somehow he found himself staring at the back of his middle finger, and it occurred to him that there might be a point there to treat the pain. He proceeded to stick his finger with the tip of a ballpoint pen and indeed found a particularly painful area. He then inserted a needle into this sensitive spot and amazingly the headache was gone (1988, 23). Dr. Yoo went on to map a representation of the body on the hand and was even able to find meridians (channels) on the hand corresponding to the body meridians. In a course on Korean hand acupuncture, I learned that because there are active acupuncture points on the hand, various things we do with our hands could actually affect our health. Stimulating acupuncture points on the hand, just as on the body, can bring about physiological changes as profound as lowering blood sugar. A serious hand injury, depending on its location, can affect a distant body part. The instructor told the story of a woman who dated the onset of an intestinal disturbance to the time of her marriage. Her hand acupuncturist found a relationship between the wedding band she was wearing and her malady. This system is quite fluid. Needles need not be the only form of stimulation. Metal pellets can be taped to the hand. Treatment can also be in the form of various types of metallic rings, rendering therapy painless and therefore useful for pediatric patients. Some acupuncturists have used diode rings to help patients with attention deficit/hyperactivity disorder. When I consider all the possible microsystems that have yet to be discovered and how intricate the body is, I can't help wondering if the body-piercing fad will have an effect on health.

How does acupuncture work?

With progress in technology, the answer to how acupuncture works is still evolving. New imaging techniques show that acupuncture actually causes functional changes in the brain and nervous system. The prevailing theory of how acupuncture works is neurohumoral. This means that the acupuncture needles send messages via the nerves to the spinal cord and to the brain where hormones are secreted. Needling acupuncture points stimulates the body to produce potent painkilling hormones called endorphins. I have often observed this endorphin-type response after the first treatment. Patients usually arise from the treatment table relaxed, and they may have even slept through the twenty-minute session. There may be an initial relief of pain, but that relief lasts only three to four hours. Some patients report feeling drowsy, and in some rare instances they may even have slight nausea. This kind of response is strikingly similar to that seen with narcotic analgesic drugs. Naloxone, a drug known to reverse the effects of narcotic painkillers, can also reverse the pain-relieving effects of acupuncture.

Patients who respond well to nonsteroidal anti-inflammatory drugs most often respond well to acupuncture. There is some evidence that needling also stimulates the pituitary gland to secrete ACTH, which in turn stimulates the adrenal gland to produce steroid hormones, known to be anti-inflammatory. There is a difference, though, between the responses to acupuncture and those to steroids. We know that when a patient whose condition responds to steroids stops the drug, the condition returns. After a course of acupuncture, however, the effect seems to be lasting. Therefore, the explanation of how acupuncture works must involve more than just its neurohumoral effect.

I was taught to feel for temperature changes on the skin to diagnose diseased areas. This simple clinical observation precludes doing expensive thermography testing, sometimes used in difficult cases to show temperature changes in diseased areas. A diseased area may be cooler than its surrounding tissue, indicating decreased circulation to the area. TCM often describes this as "blocked Qi." An inflamed area will be hotter than its surroundings. When tissue is injured or inflamed, pain-causing chemicals called cytokines accumulate. With time, the circulation will normally remove the cytokines. But if the clean-up mechanism that should normally follow inflammation is impaired or delayed, there is prolonged swelling and pain.

In general, previous steroid injections tend to diminish the effect of acupuncture. When steroids are injected into an inflamed area, the inflammation will decrease because the steroid constricts blood vessels and diminishes blood flow to the site. The downside to steroid injections, though, is that the decreased blood flow can compromise the healing process, and the injected steroid can cause muscles and tendons to become weakened, resulting in tears and ruptures. This is the reason why Western doctors put a limit on the frequency of local steroid injections. Many of my patients told me about their experiences with steroid injections. Initially the injection seemed to be effective, but when the condition recurred, subsequent injections were no longer effective. If the injection was close to the skin surface, patients often pointed out the typical cold white scar over the injection site.

In contrast to steroid injections, acupuncture increases blood flow to the area of the body being treated, and thus promotes healing. After inserting acupuncture needles, I would see the skin around the needle turn red and become warm. Acupuncture creates tiny zones of trauma, which stimulate blood flow to them. The increased blood flow helps bring nutrients to diseased areas that were previously cold and deprived of blood. TCM practitioners called it moving Qi. Acupuncture also helps hot inflamed areas by allowing the improved circulation to remove cytokines, responsible for inflammation, from tissue. When patients asked me whether they should try the steroid injection their Western doctors recommended before trying acupuncture, I usually advised them to try acupuncture first.

Some patients may have a two-phase response to acupuncture. Their pain may initially increase and then start to diminish after a day or two. During the initial worsening stage, the increased blood flow to the area may cause further congestion before the cytokines are mobilized. For other patients, the initial worsening is followed not by improvement but only by a return to their baseline pain. Their circulation may be inadequate to clear the cytokine accumulation in the tissues, and acupuncture may not be effective for them.

Does acupuncture cure or only mask pain?

Calling a treatment a cure may be a matter of semantics. The HIV-AIDS epidemic has changed our understanding of the word "cure." When the body's immune system is decimated, are there any curative antibiotics, or should we view antibiotics as a treatment that controls growth of bacteria to allow the body to conquer the invaders? Acupuncture improves the blood flow to an injured or malfunctioning area to help the body heal itself. For degenerative diseases, acupuncture neither reverses nor halts degeneration. Patients with conditions such as degenerative disc disease or degenerative arthritis who improve after the initial course of therapy do better with booster treatments at regular intervals.

Mrs. N. came to me barely able to walk even with the help of a walker. She was in agony with back and leg pain from lumbar spinal stenosis. After seven semi-weekly treatments, she improved greatly and was able to walk using just a cane. I felt gratified when I saw her strutting to the local supermarket. After a month without treatment, she returned, again a basket case. I then had to start over with weekly treatments and then space regular boosters at three-week intervals to maintain her improved state.

Another patient, Mr. A., who was seventy-three, gave a history of awakening on Thanksgiving Day with severe right leg pain. Two days later, he was doubled over in pain and walked with a limp. A CT scan showed lumbar spinal stenosis. Neither a steroid epidural nor sixteen chiropractic manipulations helped him. Four months later, when Mr. A. came to see me, he was able to walk only fifty feet and stand for only twenty minutes before pain in his leg set in. His hobby was deep-sea salmon fishing, but he was unable to continue because standing while catching fish caused pain in his leg. After four weekly treatments, Mr. A. was able to walk five blocks and remain standing for forty minutes. After eleven treatments, he went deep-sea fishing and was able to catch a thirty-pound salmon. After the fifteenth treatment, he came for a booster at monthly intervals, and he was able to bring me smoked salmon from his catch.

Is the response to acupuncture just a placebo effect?
Double-blind studies used in drug research are difficult to apply to acupuncture. Patients know whether they have been needled or not. The closest investigational method is to use sham acupuncture points. Some skeptics remain unconvinced that acupuncture therapy is effective.

Kathy, a pet hospital administrator, came to see me for treatment of her asthma. Her symptoms were quite severe, so I recommended not only acupuncture but also herbs. I gave her my routine warning about the negative aspects of herbal therapy: the time required to prepare them, the cost, and the bad taste and smell. I was surprised when she said she knew all about that. A veterinarian in her hospital used complementary care, both herbal therapy and acupuncture, for animals. She said that during high allergy season, the hospital was swamped with dogs whose owners sought acupuncture for their pets. The results were good. I asked her how they were able to keep the animals still for the treatments. Interestingly, they did it by pre-medicating the animals with a homeopathic remedy called Calming. That, along with having the owners present, seemed to work well.

The fact that response to acupuncture is as effective in animals as it is in humans would certainly argue against a placebo effect. Studies also show that during acupuncture there are measurable humoral (natural chemicals in the blood) changes and actual blood flow changes in the brain.

Do different people respond differently to acupuncture?

It did not take me long to discover that not everyone responds to acupuncture. Early in my career, my Aunt Pansy referred her close friend Jennie to me. Aunt Jennie was in her eighties and suffered from shoulder pain. When I examined her, she had typical tendonitis of the shoulder, involving the rotator cuff. She had tenderness over the location of the rotator cuff, and signs of impingement where the pain worsened when she tried to raise her arm above her head. I had treated other patients with the same problem successfully, so I readily recommended acupuncture. Desperate to find relief, Aunt Jennie agreed to try it. The morning after I treated her, Aunt Jennie called me to say her shoulder pain was even worse. I was chagrined and embarrassed at not being able to help my aunt's friend. I instructed her to ice the area and prescribed an anti-inflammatory, advising her not to get any more acupuncture. I then realized the truth of Dr. Lai's precept: acupuncture only redistributes energy. When the patient's energy is low, if not replenished, acupuncture will not be effective. Aunt Jennie, a frail octogenarian, may have had a circulatory system inadequate to the task of carrying away the pain-causing cytokines. In general, I found that older patients with multiple medical problems were less likely to respond to acupuncture. In such cases, they should be pre-treated with herbs to improve overall energy. This concept was difficult to communicate to patients, who were eager for relief and came expecting acupuncture to be their answer. Many also came with the Western purist mindset that one should try only one mode of treatment at a time in order to know which one actually helped. Convincing them to think outside the box was difficult.

Some cases are too advanced from an anatomical perspective for acupuncture to be effective. With a herniated disc or spinal stenosis, important determinants are the size of the herniation and the degree of stenosis influencing how severely the nerve root is being pinched. In spinal stenosis, the opening between two vertebrae where the nerve root emerges is narrowed. The cause may be that the disc, which is situated like a washer between the two vertebrae, has degenerated or herniated, resulting in some swelling and inflammation, blocking the opening. Acupuncture acts to widen the opening by decreasing the disc inflammation and by relaxing the tightened muscles that hold the vertebrae together. If the opening is extremely narrow, acupuncture's effect may not widen the opening enough to relieve compression of the nerve. Acupuncture has often been recommended for stroke rehabilitation. Here again, researchers have shown that the response to acupuncture depends on the size and location of the brain tissue injured. Margaret Naeser, Ph.D., found that among stroke patients with arm and leg paralysis, those who respond to acupuncture have some preserved isolated finger movement, and their brain CT scans show the size of the infarct (area of dead cells) to be less than 50 percent of the periventricular white matter (an area of the brain). Patients who have larger sized strokes did not respond to acupuncture (Naeser 1996).

When I am asked whether acupuncture is effective for a particular condition, I no longer give a glib general answer. Cases often need to be individualized. The sharing of experiences by acupuncturists and further research can offer important and useful guidelines.

Conditions Treatable with Acupuncture

Whenever patients came to me seeking acupuncture, I relied on my Western understanding of their disease process. I required that patients either have a primary physician overseeing their care, or at least have a Western diagnosis. There is evidence that about 80 percent of patients who respond to acupuncture begin to improve within three treatments. With this in mind, I would then proceed without initial expensive tests. If, after the initial three treatments, there was no improvement, there was still time to order tests. If the patient's condition began to improve, further testing was not needed. Often, with our Western mindset, we do not think immediately of acupuncture as a viable option when first presented with a malady. Over the years, I have found that there are some common conditions for which acupuncture has proven to be a good first option.

Musculoskeletal Pain

Soft tissue injuries and inflammation such as cervical and lumbar disc disease, tendonitis, tennis elbow, plantar fasciitis, carpal tunnel syndrome, and tension headaches all respond well to acupuncture. In my acupuncture practice, treating back pain was about as common as treating colds. The earlier I began treatment, the more rapid the response. If I treated a young robust patient with a recent back injury, he or she was usually able to return to work within a week, and the symptoms completely resolved in a matter of three weeks. Such acute cases responded far more quickly than chronic back pain cases because the vicious cycle of pain and muscle tightening had not yet set in. When there is pain, the muscles tighten to splint the diseased area, causing more pain and further muscle tightening.

For muscle spasm, acupuncture may work in two ways. The needling improves circulation to the muscles and causes them to relax. Needling muscles also initiates a reflex cycle of contraction followed by relaxation (Gunn 1997, 109–112) This phenomenon is similar to what happens when the doctor taps the knee to evaluate reflexes while the patient is in a sitting position. When struck at the knee tendon, the thigh muscles contract, causing the knee to pop out in extension. What naturally follows is a relaxation of the thigh muscle causing the knee to then fall back down into the resting flexed position. The technique called Intramuscular Stimulation (IMS), originated by Chan Gunn, M.D., is directed at needling tense muscles. I trained in it in Canada and found it very effective, but when I tried to use it in the United States, I found that my American patients were not such willing subjects because the technique is more painful than conventional acupuncture. I therefore used a modification of it. Instead of needling multiple tight muscles many times to achieve the relaxation, I directed one needle to an area of muscle tightness and used electrical stimulation to enhance spreading of the stimulation.

An interesting aside is that Dr. Gunn taught that unilateral tinea pedis (a fungal infection known as athlete's foot) often responded to needling at the lumbar spine. He explained that when nerves emerging from the lumbar spine are pinched, the nervous and circulatory flow to the feet are diminished, and that leads to lowered immunity to the fungus. With needling, pressure to the nerve is relieved and blood flow becomes normalized. As a result, skin immunity of the foot on that side is restored. I had a patient who complained of lumbar back pain with sciatica. I treated her back problem with acupuncture and witnessed fulfillment of

Dr. Gunn's prediction. When her back pain was relieved, she told me that the longstanding fungus skin infection of the foot on that same side also cleared.

Recently, allopathic medicine has been rethinking the origin of arthritis. Perhaps arthritic pain begins with muscle tightening. Joints are the interface between two bones insulated by cartilage, connected by ligaments, and held together by muscles. It is possible that joint inflammation actually begins when the muscles around the joint tighten, causing more friction between the cartilages covering the two bones. Part of the effect of acupuncture is to relax the muscles surrounding joints thereby reducing this friction.

Reports have emerged showing that the drug Botox, derived from Botulinum toxin, which causes muscle paralysis, can be injected into back muscles to reduce pain. Actually, acupuncture needles have been achieving the same effect for thousands of years at far less cost. Another recent study looked at Botox's effect on the flexion contracture of wrist and hand muscles in stroke victims (Brashear, et al. 2002). With a stroke, the brain's function of balancing flexion and extension of limbs is lost, and the stronger flexor muscles become dominant. Botox was injected to see if the flexor muscles could be relaxed to normalize the limbs. The study showed improvement not only in the Botox subjects but some improvement in the placebo subjects as well. A plausible explanation for the response in the placebo subjects is that their muscles were poked with needles while receiving the placebo injections. Those needles, to some degree, caused the muscles to go through contraction followed by relaxation.

Upper and Lower Respiratory Problems

My later experience with acupuncture taught me the importance of keeping an open mind. On my first day in ACTCM class, when the instructor suggested that sinusitis could be cured with acupuncture and herbs, I scoffed. Since then, I have used acupuncture frequently to help reverse congestion in both the nose and the eustachian tubes. People frequently travel by air with nasal congestion caused by either colds or nasal allergies. Upon the plane's descent, the passenger feels pressure or pain in his or her ears because the eustachian tubes, which normally equalize air pressure between the ears and the outside atmosphere, are constricted from swelling in their walls. The same process that causes a stuffy nose with colds or allergies occurs in the eustachian tubes. After the flight, the unequalized pressure in the eustachian tubes can cause the patient to feel as if the ears are plugged for a long time. Acupuncture enhances blood flow to the eustachian tubes and thereby reduces the congestion and widens the passageways.

When treating nasal allergies, I used a similar technique to open up the nasal passages and added immune-boosting acupuncture points such as LI 4 and St 36 (Joos, et al. 2000). To treat asthma, I have used similar points coupled with points that enhance breathing, such as Lu 7 and UB 13. These points lower Qi and likely dilate bronchial tubes. In most of these cases, my therapy also included herbs to replenish energy.

Autonomic Dysfunctions

The autonomic nervous system, responsible for controlling so many internal organ functions, can often be regulated using acupuncture. One physician acupuncturist colleague told me long ago that he had successfully used acupuncture to treat pancreatitis. Usually the points used in these treatments are remote from the organ, and the remoteness of the points has promulgated an aura of mystery around this Eastern approach. I believe that there is a scientific explanation. When I trained in anesthesiology, I was taught that to perform spinal anesthesia for knee surgery, we needed to block the nerves not only up to a level where the sensory nerves to the knee emanate from the spinal cord but to a much higher level. This is because there are some sympathetic nerve fibers running along the peripheral nerves to the knee, and if the spinal anesthetic missed those nerves as they emerged from the spinal cord at a higher level, the patient would have pain during surgery. Many acupuncture points are located on peripheral nerves. It is probable that there are autonomic nerves accompanying these peripheral nerves, not completely mapped out in our anatomy books. This could explain why acupuncturing points on the limbs influence heart rate, bowel motility, and uterine contractions. With conditions involving organ dysfunction, such as irritable bowel or constipation, acupuncture stimulates the nerves supplying the area in order to normalize the function. In contrast, Western drugs act unidirectionally; one drug is used to slow down intestinal motility when it is too fast, and another drug is used to stimulate the bowel when it is too slow.

Scar Tissue

Treating scar tissue using Western methods poses a challenge. With reoperation, the trauma of the surgery often leads to further scarring. Steroid injections help sometimes, but not always. Acupuncture, by the same mechanism of improving blood flow to an area, can successfully shrink scar tissue. Mr. W., age seventy-five, had right knee pain for three years following a freak accident when he fell on an open knife, lacerating that knee. The laceration was sutured, but the wound re-bled, and required re-suturing. Since then, Mr. W. had suffered from chronic right knee and right hip pain. Sharp jabbing pains, beginning in the knee and radiating up his thigh, often punctuated the chronic pain. He walked with a limp. Mr. W. underwent arthroscopic exploration seven months before consulting with me, but his symptoms had not improved with this procedure. I felt that the jabbing pain was caused by scar tissue, and I acupunctured his scar as well as the knee joint, hip joint, and lower back. After ten treatments, Mr. W. greatly improved and was able to walk ten blocks. Seven months after beginning treatment, he was able to walk three miles without pain, and the spontaneous jabbing pains disappeared. He then was maintained on monthly therapy.

Another patient, Mr. L., age fifty-five, had undergone a vasectomy. The surgery was complicated by an infection, causing pain in his right groin. The surgeon reoperated and removed a granuloma (an excessive growth of tissue the body forms to isolate foreign material commonly seen as a reaction to splinters). After the second surgery, Mr. L. continued to have pain in his right groin, which was tender when it was bumped; the pain worsened after intercourse. I treated with weekly acupuncture, and the pain resolved after about eight months of treatment. It occasionally recurred, but one or two booster acupuncture treatments easily controlled it.

Headaches

Treating vascular headaches such as migraines has been challenging. The classic explanation of how these headaches develop is that there is an inherent instability in the blood vessels in the brains of migraine sufferers. When there is a temporary decrease in blood flow to the brain because of this instability, a message is sent to the heart to pump more blood to the head. The increased blood flow to the scalp is what causes the headache. Drugs that specifically constrict this reflexive increase in blood flow are sometimes effective for treatment. In my experience with acupuncture, using classic points recommended in textbooks has not been very successful. In later years, if a patient's headaches responded to sumatriptin, a drug specific for vascular headaches, I would not consider treating him or her with acupuncture.

Robert, the husband of one of my patients, was such a case. Robert's wife told me he was suffering from severe cluster headaches, and was taking sumatriptin as regularly as vitamins. I told her that I doubted if I could help him. Despite my gloomy forecast, one day, in desperation, he came to see me. He said that his symptoms were related to the weather. They were much worse during the rainy season. During the drought we had in San Francisco, he was headache-free. He found sumatriptin helped, but he became dependent on it. When I examined him, the muscles in his neck were extremely tense. It then occurred to me that the worsening of his symptoms during rainy weather might be similar to the phenomenon seen among arthritics who can sense when it will rain more accurately than the meteorologists. I wondered if his neck muscle tension might be an accompaniment of some degree of degenerative cervical disc disease. When I acupunctured the tense muscles and advised Robert to improve the ergonomics at his computer workstation, his headaches resolved and he stopped taking sumatriptin. My experience with his case has taught me that not all vascular headaches are purely vascular in origin. If there is a muscle tension component to the headache, I have found acupuncture can help. In a 2002 issue of *Time* magazine devoted to headaches, the authors, quoting research findings, also suggest that the prevailing explanation for migraines may be too simplistic (Gorman and Park 2002, 79–82). Headaches may result from many factors.

Reflex Sympathetic Dystrophy

Carrie, in her thirties, sustained a severe hand injury while water-skiing. Some bones were broken and some tendons were severed. After multiple surgeries, she suffered from chronic pain accompanied by coldness and pallor in her hand called sympathetic dystrophy (also known as causalgia). In these cases, there is an excessive sympathetic response to the injury. The blood vessels to the injured area constrict, resulting in diminished blood flow to the area, a very difficult condition to treat. I acupunctured a point in the armpit (Ht 1) in the location of the brachial plexus and points (Baxie) between her fingers where the interdigital nerves emerge. With the treatments, her hand warmed up. In the past, as an anesthesiologist, I used to inject local anesthetic into these points to numb the nerves to the hand or fingers for surgery. For this condition, I did not need to inject a drug. Just needling the points proved very effective. Since treating Carrie, I have used this approach successfully on other patients with reflex sympathetic dystrophy.

Reproductive Tract Disorders

One of my first successes while still a student at ACTCM was using acupuncture to treat an ER co-worker's epididymitis. In my integrated practice, there were many more women than men seeking acupuncture for reproductive tract disorders. Perhaps it is because information about acupuncture has been more widely publicized for women's health than for male reproductive problems. Nevertheless, I believe acupuncture is effective in treating reproductive tract problems of both genders. I have treated many cases of menstrual pain, female infertility, and the pain from endometriosis, a condition where the lining of the uterus somehow is implanted outside the uterus. In fact, whenever a member of my office staff had menstrual pain, I would acupuncture her and get her back to work with full relief within a half hour.

There is a point on the medial aspect of the lower leg, San Yin Jiao (Spleen 6), that I used frequently to treat reproductive tract disorders. The location of the point is actually on the path of the posterior tibial nerve. One day I used this point to treat a leg condition. After I inserted the needle, the patient exclaimed that she felt the sensation in her genital area. Urologists have successfully used electrical stimulation of this same point, Spleen 6, to treat urinary bladder dysfunction (Klinger, et al. 2000; Mc Guire 1983). The posterior tibial nerve actually is a nerve supplying the muscles to the leg and foot. How can it affect the genitourinary tract? The genitourinary tract is supplied by the pudendal nerve, which shares the nerve roots S2 and S3 with the posterior tibial nerve. Urology researchers believe that stimulating the posterior tibial nerve sends an antidromic impulse (going in a direction opposite to the normal) up to the S3 nerve root, which then travels down the pudendal nerve (Mc Guire 1983). Antidromal nerve conduction is another explanation of how stimulating distant acupuncture points can affect internal organs.

Acupuncture in a Third-World Setting

Medical missions have been my passion ever since I became a Christian while an undergraduate at the University of California, Berkeley. I participated in many projects in various parts of the world, including Taiwan, Macao, Xinjiang, and Yunnan, China. My frustration was seeing a need but not being able to meet it with Western medicine. Without the infrastructure I was accustomed to, I could not apply what I did as a Western practitioner to situations in impoverished countries. When taking a history to diagnose diseases of the colon, I was taught to ask the patients what their stools looked like: were there any tarry or any pencil-slim stools, and so forth. How was I to do that when people use outhouses? Many Western diagnoses are based on laboratory tests. Many places I visited had no labs.

When I heard that there would be a new opportunity to do medical mission work in a town called Tokmok in Kyrgyzstan, and that the clinic soon to be opened would be providing acupuncture as one of the services, I volunteered to go. I first went to observe the building of the clinic in the year 2000, and subsequently returned for six- to eight-week stints in 2001 and 2002.

Kyrgyzstan is in Central Asia. To its north is the oil rich country of Kazakhstan. To its southeast, the beautiful snowcapped Tian Shan (Heavenly Mountain) range separates it from Xinjiang, China. Directly south, Tajikistan separates it from Afghanistan. And to its west, is Uzbekistan, whose city, Samarkand, was depicted in the *Arabian Nights*. It was part of the Soviet Union until its dissolution in 1991.

The population is made up of occidental Russians; Central Asians from Kyrgyz; Uzbek and Tajik tribes; and Dungan people, who are originally from the Chinese provinces of Shanxi and Gansu. Their ancestry can be traced to mixed marriages between Arab Silk Road traders and the Hui inhabitants of these two provinces.

The Qing dynasty emperor ordered them to leave China because he suspected this mixed-race Muslim group of being insurrectionists. They fled westward, crossing the formidable Tian Shan mountain range. Survivors of this arduous migration settled in Kazakhstan and Kyrgyzstan.

In affluent Western countries, fast foods and physical inactivity have led to the diseases of diabetes, obesity, and hypertension. In Central Asia, the same diseases are prevalent, but the source is different. The people's high consumption of carbohydrates and saturated fats is a habit originating from their past nomadic lifestyle. Many raised sheep and ate lamb. A family of modest means once invited me to lunch. From the taste, I could tell that the rice pilaf served was cooked in mutton fat. Harsh winters required the people to preserve fruits and vegetables. Bread and jam became common staples. Tea is commonly sweetened with jam. Whenever I made a house call, I was regularly invited to sit at the family's low dining table situated on a platform, and have tea with jam before leaving. While diseases in Central Asians are the same as those commonly seen in the West, the lack of resources in this region of the world dictated a paradigm shift in order to treat them. Because of their cultural mix, the people of this region proved to be receptive to Eastern health remedies, and they readily accepted acupuncture.

Luke Services International bought a large restaurant that had gone out of business and converted it into the Hope Clinic. Some of the walls did not extend all the way up to the ceiling, and some of the rooms had mirrors on the ceiling. To avoid providing a strip show, we had to be careful which rooms to use when examining patients.

At the clinic, there were two permanent full-time Russian physicians. Nadia was a cardiologist who spoke English, and Katia was a retired pediatrician. I served mainly as the clinic acupuncturist. With so few resources, I found acupuncture very useful and began employing it in ways I had never imagined before.

Hot Flashes

Barbara was forty-three and teaching English in Kyrgyzstan. She had missed about three periods and was suffering from severe hot flashes. Ventilation was poor in the room where she held classes, and the temperature was about 90 degrees F. Even before the many negative research studies surfaced, I was never a proponent of routine estrogen replacement. For extreme symptoms such as Barbara's, however, I have prescribed it for short-term relief. I advised her to inquire about hormone replacement therapy when she returned to the United States. Barbara said that Nadia had prescribed a local plant estrogen formula for her, which helped some, but it failed to bring adequate relief. Synthetic estrogens were unavailable locally. Having very little to lose, I decided to treat Barbara with acupuncture, using the Endocrine point on her ear. The results were dramatic. The next morning, she reported she was able to sleep through the entire night without a single hot flash awakening her. In her classroom, the students noticed that she no longer needed to use a stack of paper towels to wipe off her perspiration.

On one of the hottest days of the year, Barbara, our local guide, Misha, and I went to the museum in Bishkek, the capital city. I found the heat overpowering. Misha, who was a native, commented that even he found the heat on that July day unbearable. Barbara said, "I don't know what you two are talking about. I feel just comfortable." Her comment made me decide to cut back on the frequency of her treatments from daily to three times a week. At the end of six weeks, Barbara finally had a period, the first in three months. Two years later, and back in the United States, I was in contact with her. Her periods had returned to near normal, and her hot flashes were gone. For Barbara, acupuncturing the Ear Endocrine point was effective because her ovaries still retained function. For older women, further into menopause, stimulating weaker ovaries might not be as effective.

Menstrual Irregularity

Olga, a patient in her forties, had metrorrhagia (abnormally frequent menstrual bleeding). She was bleeding almost constantly through-out the month. I asked about her Pap smear and endometrial biopsy. Nadia assured me that Olga had had a gynecologic workup that ruled out cancer as a cause of the bleeding. In the United States, the treatment would be to prescribe hormones, often in the form of birth control pills, to regulate her bleeding quickly. With my integrated practice, I used herbs as well to improve circulation to the ovaries and stabilize the patient's own hormones. With neither of these options available in Kyrgyzstan, I also ventured to treat Olga with acupuncture, using the Endocrine ear point. Remarkably, after two weekly treatments, Olga's bleeding ceased.

Blocked Tear Duct

On another occasion, Barbara told me she suffered from tearing in one eye. I figured she had a blocked tear duct on that side. If we had been in the United States, I would have sent her to an oph-thalmologist who could insert a probe into the tear duct to clear the obstruction, but that option was not available. I thought about the anatomy of the tear duct, which dives from the inner corner of the eye into the nose. There is an acupuncture point called Bitong, meaning "clear the nose," which is located near the bridge of the nose along the path of the tear duct. I decided to acupuncture that point to improve circulation to the tear duct area and allow it to open up, as I had done so often with eustachian tube blockages. I did it, and advised Barbara to drink plenty of fluids to encourage liquefying the contents plugging her tear duct. After one treatment, the tearing stopped, and Barbara became an even more ardent believer in acupuncture with both her maladies remedied.

Varicose Veins

Using acupuncture to treat varicose veins never crossed my mind until my trip to Kyrgyzstan, where the patients begged me to treat them. They were enthusiastic because another physician-acupuncturist who preceded me had treated varicose veins with good results. I was skeptical. My understanding of varicose veins was that the one-way valves in the leg veins leak because they are weak and do not close completely, that this was an irreversible structural condition, usually hereditary, and that the only solution was mechanical. You could either strip the leaky veins for cosmetic reasons, or use elastic stockings as a source of external pressure to assist the blood flow in the leg veins. At the urging of my local colleague, Nadia, who had witnessed the good results with acupuncture, I agreed to try. To my surprise, within three weeks I was able to help a patient with a varicose ulcer heal by using acupuncture. Even more astounding was that a patient whom I was treating with acupuncture for lower back pain pointed out that when his back improved, so did his varicose veins.

I rethought the matter and considered that perhaps weak, loose valves are not the only factor causing varicose veins. When I returned home to my anatomy books, I read that nerves supply veins just as they do arteries, but that the number of nerves supplying veins is fewer than those to arteries. If the vein walls are under nervous control, they can dilate and constrict similar to the way arteries change size. When the nerves to those veins are pinched or not functioning normally, as occurs with lumbar disc disease, the veins lose normal tone. Acupuncture for lumbar disc disease improves the vitality of the nerve supply to the leg veins and, therefore, restores venous wall tone. TCM practitioners would say that the acupuncture functioned to move Qi. I related my experience to Dr. Lai, and he said he commonly used acupuncture to treat varicose veins.

Nadia and I often compared notes on various subjects. She found varicose veins and varicose ulcers very common at Hope Clinic. I agreed with her but said I found the condition far more common among Russian patients than Kyrgyz or Dungan patients. Could it be because of the differences in their habits? Varicose veins and varicose ulcers result from the inability of the blood supplying the legs and feet to return to the heart adequately. The backed-up blood increases the pressure in the leg veins, causing them to bulge. The increased pressure also causes seepage of some blood out of the vein into the skin layer where iron from red blood cells deposits, causing ugly discoloration, and eventually the skin breaks down, forming varicose ulcers. The tendency for the blood to back up in the leg veins is worsened by gravity when the legs are in a dependent position such as with sitting or standing. Western habits such as that of sitting at a desk, using a toilet, and sitting at a dining table all tend to worsen varicose veins. Kyrgyz and Dungan people, like the Japanese, by contrast, ate at low tables sitting on the floor. The pressure in their leg veins was lower than that in their Russian counterparts, who sat on chairs with their legs in the dependent position much of the time. In addition, Kyrgyz and Dungan toilets were at ground level, requiring them to squat, a position that also reduces leg vein pressure. Nadia concurred. She had never seen the condition in these two ethnic groups. She pointed out an additional factor: they habitually prostrate them-selves to pray to Allah five times a day. This posture also relieves leg vein pressure.

Burn Wound

One day, while I was treating a young Dungan woman for lumbar disc disease, my nurse, Sonia, noticed that the patient had a fresh burn on both buttocks. Perhaps because of modesty, the patient never mentioned it. She had fallen backwards into a tub of hot water. The diameter of the burn area was about 4.5 cm on each side. The location must have made urination and defecation very painful and uncomfortable. The clinic did not even have Silvadene, an antibiotic ointment for burns. Extrapolating from my experience treating varicose ulcers, I reasoned that perhaps acupuncturing around the burn site would accelerate healing by increasing blood flow to the area. I asked the patient to come daily, and I needled circumferentially around her burn wounds. The areas healed in two weeks with no infection.

Meralgia Paresthetica

One of my successful experiences was with a patient who had meralgia paresthetica, a condition in which there is a well-defined area of numbness, about the size of a hand, in the front of the thigh. It is usually caused by compression of the lateral femoral cutaneous nerve as it emerges from the pelvis on the way to the thigh. The compression might result from excessively tight clothing or wearing objects that rest on the area where the nerve is. In the United States, I treated a meter maid who hung her phone from the waist, leading to compression of the area. With this patient in Kyrgyzstan, the cause was not completely clear because I could not get a very detailed history, but her symptoms were easy to diagnose. The treatment is to needle around the area where the nerve emerges. The acupuncture stimulates circulation to the area, taking away the tissue edema around the nerve. In my experience, treatment for this condition is simple and very effective.

Ankle Pain from an Old Injury

The mother of Masha, one of the nurses at the clinic, had broken her leg three times in the past. She had chronic ankle pain, and usually she could hardly walk by evening. Her ankle appeared quite deformed. I treated her ankle by needling where I thought the tendons and ligaments were strained excessively by the altered mechanics of walking. At the end of my stay, she asked Nadia to tell me in English that she was grateful because she was able to put in a full day's work. She raised cows, as did many of the locals there. Usually, about five families would take turns cow sitting for each other. One person would watch all the cows, about twenty in all, as they grazed. Before her treatments, Masha's mom could never take part in her neighborhood's cow-sitting pool, but now she was a happy participant.

Ankylosing Spondylitis

One day Nadia told me that a man in his early thirties would be coming from a distant village to see me because of spine and chest pain. She suspected a condition called ankylosing spondylitis, an autoimmune disease that causes gradual fusion with consequent stiffness of the spine. I asked if his blood had tested positive for the HLA-B27 antigen commonly found in patients with this condition. She told me the test was unavailable. When I saw the patient, Sasha, he indeed seemed to have the condition. He had kyphosis (hunching) of his thoracic spine, pain along most of the length of his spine, and rib pain. I remembered treating one other case in the United States, without success, and was reluctant to try. Nadia said, "You have to try; you're his only hope." Under these circumstances, I agreed to try. I was surprised that after the first treatment, Sasha's rib pain disappeared; after three treatments, although his bent-over condition had not improved, he had good pain relief. After Sasha's four treatments, my time at Hope Clinic ended. I hoped I had taught Nadia enough to continue treating Sasha.

In Kyrgyzstan, with its ethnic diversity, I felt it easy to blend in. I was especially pleased when one day a Russian woman stopped me to ask for directions to the Umeda Café, which was the café next to the condominium where I was staying. I was able to tell her in my limited Russian, learned at San Francisco State University, "It's not far. Just walk two blocks and it will be on your left." She thanked me, and I felt proud of my Russian fluency and for being mistaken for a local. Kyrgyzstan is on the Silk Road, which has come to mean the path where Eastern and Western cultures intersect. I brought back with me an understanding that in a part of the world where expensive Western medical resources are unavailable, an ancient Eastern remedy, acupuncture, can benefit many people.

Chapter 11

The TCM View of Diet

In the course of my practice, I was struck by the difference between the Western and Eastern concepts of what comprises a healthy diet. Many young women in their reproductive years, with a Western outlook, told me that their diets consisted mainly of salads and very little meat. They were proud of "eating healthy." For them, this meant high fiber, low fat, and low calories. From the Eastern perspective, this diet is not considered healthful for young women.

TCM teaches that because of menstrual blood loss, women in their reproductive years tend to be Blood 血 and Yang 陽 Deficient 虛, putting them in a Cold 寒 state. Their intake of food or herbs should be warming and tonifying to blood. Meats, which are considered warm, are more suitable for them than salads, which are categorized as cool. Arteriosclerosis and hypertensive heart disease are Yang conditions, usually more prevalent in males in midlife. For them, cool salads and meat reduction are in order. A woman in her reproductive years, however, is at low risk for this type of Yang condition. Unbalanced overconsumption of leafy vegetables, which are categorized as cool, is inappropriate for young women because it tends to magnify an existing Cold condition.

In 1989, on the day of the Loma Prieta earthquake in San Francisco, a young woman came to see me because of a persistent allergic skin condition. She gave a history of having been a vegetarian and a blood donor. My impression was that she was Yang and Blood deficient, so I advised her to stop donating blood and incorporate complete proteins such as poultry, meat, and fish into her diet. In the middle of our consultation the earthquake struck. It must have reinforced my message. She called me a while later to say she had taken my advice and her skin condition had resolved.

Another woman, also a vegetarian in her thirties, came to see me for pain in her spine. Four months before, she had fallen down some stairs with her infant baby in her arms. As a result, she sustained a fracture of her eighth thoracic vertebra. Fortunately, the baby was unhurt, but after the fall, my patient suffered from persistent pain and numbness at the site of the fracture. She had just quit her job, and she was breast-feeding her baby. I told her she was on the right track by quitting her job, thereby sparing her energy. I advised her to gradually add meat to her diet. With the change in her habits, and after seven acupuncture sessions, her symptoms resolved.

Influenced by their TCM heritage, Chinese patients customarily regard food and medicine as interchangeable. When they ask their Western physicians to advise them about diet, they are really asking about how best to balance their own deficiencies or excesses through choice of foods. The Western physician can advise about diet for some conditions: for diabetes, limit the glucose and simple carbohydrate intake; for heart disease and cancer prevention, increase fiber and antioxidant-rich foods, and avoid saturated fats. For many other conditions, though, there are no specific dietary recommendations from the Western perspective. In such cases, the physician would answer, "It doesn't matter. You can eat anything." The Chinese patient walks away disappointed. Without realizing it, doctor and patient are speaking from two very different paradigms.

Classifying people by type is common in most cultures. The Greeks have categories such as sanguine and phlegmatic. The Chinese classify not only people and disease types but also food types. Almost all foods fall into one or more TCM categories. Normally, foods are combined in such a way as to balance each other to neutrality. For example, leafy green vegetables, known to be cold, are often cooked with ginger, which is spicy and hot, to create balance. Meats, which are considered Yang, are sautéed with vegetables, which are considered Yin.

The cuisines of other countries also reflect this instinctive tendency toward balance. In French cuisine, buttery dishes, high in fat content, are balanced with garlic and onions, which tend to disperse and neutralize fats, thus discouraging harmful arteriosclerosis plaques from forming. Europeans also drink red wine, which neutralizes some of the harmful effects of the fats in their diet.

Environment is another factor in the TCM choice of foods. The Chinese, and probably other nationalities as well, prepare foods according to the season, with the thought of balancing the potentially detrimental effects of climate changes. In cold weather, more warming foods are eaten. In warm weather, we eat more cooling foods. Foods are also used therapeutically for their warming or cooling properties to balance a deficiency or excess in the host.

Toxic 毒 Foods

Over thousands of years, the Chinese have empirically found some foods to be less conducive to good health than others. They categorize these foods as toxic. In certain cases, these ancient beliefs have been validated by modern research. For patients whose total energy might be compromised, such as those with cancer, allergic conditions, painful arthritis, or those who recently underwent surgery, a TCM physician would counsel them to avoid certain foods considered toxic. The most common toxic food is shellfish. Interestingly, ancient Jewish dietary laws also proscribed shellfish. Modern science has discovered small amounts of arsenic in shellfish.

The other two foods in this toxic category are turkey and duck. Many Americans on low cholesterol diets have made turkey their meat of choice. I have to wonder if they are trading a benefit for a risk. Science has not yet found the basis for the Chinese belief in the toxic nature of turkey meat, so I refrain from commenting on this practice. Deep down though, I have reservations about whether turkey is the ideal meat touted by many. On the day after Thanksgiving, my grandmother used to make bitter melon soup for the family to counteract the toxic effect of the turkey consumed the previous day. Bitter melon is cool and has a cleansing toxin 解毒 property. The term "cleansing toxin" can mean antibacterial, antiviral, or anti-inflammatory.

TCM's dictum is to avoid or minimize toxic foods when the body is under excessive stress. If we consider the concept of economics of energy (see chapter 7), this makes sense. For patients with conditions that drain energy, such as wound healing or cancer, eating foods that contain anything requiring detoxification by the liver puts an extra demand on the body's energy resources.

Energy Foods

For patients who are in a Deficient state, certain foods can restore energy. TCM considers the meat of animals that exhibit high energy to be a good source. Frogs' legs are known to be the prime choice. The Chinese often prepare them for friends and family recovering from surgery or other medical conditions that deplete energy. Other meats in this category are lamb, beef, and venison.

Wet-Hot 濕熱 Foods

Mothers generally warn their children against eating too much candy or ice cream. Chinese mothers have an additional warning for their children—avoid too much Wet-Hot foods. I used to puzzle over why my mother warned me not to eat too many mangoes. This fruit is widely known among Chinese to be in the Wet-Hot category. I finally understood the meaning of this warning when I read that the allergen urushiol, found in poison ivy, is present in the skin of mangos. For people allergic to uroshiol, touching mango skin could set up a reaction similar to the one seen with poison ivy. The skin would get red and itchy; this is the "Hot" reaction. Blisters can form and often break and weep; this is the "Wet" reaction. If we keep in mind that TCM categorizations are based on observation, we can better understand the origins of the Wet-Hot category. The ancients may have observed that after ingesting certain foods, some people developed an allergic-type reaction, which, in TCM, is Wet (see chapter 4). With other foods, especially acidic fruits, certain other people might have an exacerbation of their arthritis, also known in TCM as Wind Wet (see chapter 4). So the general recommendation familiar to most Chinese is to avoid Wet-Hot foods if one has a Wet or Hot condition such as arthritis, allergic conditions, boils, or open wounds. In the absence of a Wet or Hot condition, these foods are not prohibited but should be consumed in moderation. Pineapple, mango, cherry, and strawberry fall into the Wet-Hot category. When advising patients, I used to be ambivalent about these foods. In the Western sense, they provide fiber and contain antioxidants and are considered virtuous, but from my Chinese cultural tradition, they have this Wet-Hot villainous side. I now think that these fruits have probably been unfairly maligned by generations of Chinese. My hunch is that in the absence of an allergy to them or an arthritic condition, they can be consumed with impunity. We need not feel the same guilt when eating them as when eating chocolates.

Hot 熱 or Fire 火 Qi 氣

A familiar term in Chinese folk medicine is Hot 熱 (Cantonese) or Fire 火 (Mandarin) Qi. It describes a state comprised of a constellation of ailments: acne, constipation, halitosis, dry mouth, nosebleeds, and sore throat. People with this condition are in a state of excess Yang

Heat and deficient Yin. The condition can result from a number of causes. A common one is eating hot spicy foods. For me, curry will do it. A Korean couple who had more than the normal share of sore throats and styes came often to see me as patients. As we talked, I discovered that their diet included many spicy hot foods such as Kimchi. I advised them to eat less of that type of food, and the conditions that used to plague them became less frequent.

Another less commonly recognized cause of Hot Qi is taking certain drugs. Early in my practice, I prescribed a blood pressure drug for a Chinese patient. On her follow-up visit, she complained that the drug had caused her to have Hot Qi. Her symptoms were dry mouth and constipation. At the time, I was puzzled. I had never heard of drug side effects described as Hot Qi. Later, I recognized that many drugs do have a drying effect. The list includes antihistamines for allergies and the common cold, antidepressants, drugs to treat motion sickness (meclizine in the tablet form and scopolamine in the transdermal form are two common ones), and some blood pressure medications. They will cause constipation and a dry mouth. These side effects are symptoms of Hot Qi.

Traditionally, the Chinese know how to remedy their own Hot Qi conditions by eating cool 涼, Yin-promoting 養陰 foods. A slightly more severe form of Hot Qi might be manifested by a sore throat. The mucous secretions in the mouth and throat are supplied with antibodies to fend off invading viruses and bacteria. When these secretions dry up, the immune defense mechanism declines, and the result can be a viral or even a bacterial throat infection. For mild sore throats, sometimes eating Yin-promoting foods is enough to resolve the symptoms. A more severe sore throat may indicate that an invading organism has breached the immune defense in the throat and clearing-Heat 清熱 type herbs are needed. Incidentally, sore throat is the first warning sign of a decline in white blood cell count, a side effect of some drugs such as propylthiouracil for hyperthyroidism. The significance is the same: the normal immune mechanism has been breached.

In advanced Hot Qi states, when the secretions from various glands become dry and thick, there can be an obstruction to flow, resulting in acne or styes. This again might require a little more intervention than just a change in the diet. Along this continuum, an advanced stage might be severe constipation, leading to fecolith formation, as in the case of the boy I saw in the ER who developed appendicitis (see chapter 6).

Hot Qi foods include any kind of chips, popcorn, most nuts, and most spices, especially if the flavor is spicy hot. Cooking can move a food from neutral into the Hot Qi category. Any fried or barbecued food is considered to have Hot Qi. Chocolate is also a Hot Qi food. People who already have Hot Qi symptoms, such as acne, boils, constipation, and the like, should avoid these foods. In winter, the drying effect of cold air on mucous membranes often leads to symptoms like nosebleeds and sore throats. During this season, consumption of Hot Qi foods should be minimized. The Western custom of drinking hot chocolate on a cold wintry day is antithetical to the Eastern concept of an appropriate dietary habit. According to the TCM paradigm, frosty weather is the time to avoid chocolate.

Warming 溫 Foods

While some foods, such as fried foods and chips, are always considered unhealthy because they are in the Hot Qi category, not all Warm or Hot foods are considered bad. Sometimes Hot foods are used for their warming therapeutic properties. Many spices, such as cinnamon, pepper, and ginger, are considered warming. They seem to increase blood flow and may stimulate the immune response. Most meats are also considered warming. The Warming foods are therapeutic in the early stages of a viral infection when the body feels cold intolerance or chilly, but they are not so helpful later when there is fever and inflammation. Warming foods are useful in cool states such as during menses; when there is blood loss; during the convalescent phase of an illness; and when conditions such as diminished energy, slow metabolism, and poor circulation associated with aging exist.

Warming foods are also useful with arthritic conditions, which TCM classifies as Wind and Wet. TCM also describes arthritis as a Bi 筆, or an obstructed Qi, condition. In Western terms, we might think of it as poor circulation accompanying joint stiffness. Treatment calls for warming the patient, quelling Wind, and moving Blood and Qi. In essence, the goal is to improve circulation. Besides having a warming property, some foods in the warming category also quell Wind 驅風 and dry Wet 去濕. Ginger, often taken by Chinese arthritics, is a prime example. Ginger is also widely used for nausea and gas. Studies show that it is as effective as any drug for that purpose (Micklefield, et al. 1999). In such cases, gas corresponds to the TCM term Wind, and the increased salivation and gastric secretion accompanying nausea correspond to the TCM term Wet.

My friend Ann, born in China in the 1920s before antibiotics had been discovered, told me that as an infant she became ill from a Heat disease, most likely an infectious disease. Her parents took her to see an herbalist who prescribed clearing Heat 清熱 and cleaning toxin 解毒 herbs, which are all categorized as cold. After she was given the cold herbs, her condition swung over to a very Cold state. Her parents later told her that she became pale, cold, and unresponsive, and her eyes became glazed. They presumed that she must have received an overdose of the cold herbs. Her Cold condition was so severe that the family gave up on her, but her grandfather came to the rescue. He boiled shaved cinnamon bark 肉桂 in water for her. After a teaspoonful, her parents said that life returned to her eyes, and after another, she began to look around. An interesting aside is that Ann has a Proustian aversion to the taste of cinnamon.

Cool 涼 Foods

Most leafy green vegetables, green beans, carrots, celery, and cilantro are cool foods. Some fruits such as banana, pear, and watermelon also fall into the cool category. These foods are recommended for excess Yang conditions like acne. For women who get acne before their periods, a soup of carrots, barley, and cilantro can help. A steady diet of predominantly Cool foods, though, can move a young woman into an excessively Cold state.

A young Chinese woman shared with me an experience she had. While living in Hong Kong, her diet for several months consisted mainly of vegetable soup. During that time, she developed prolonged and heavy periods to the point that she had to be hospitalized for anemia. Western-trained physicians were at a loss as to how to treat her. Finally, a Chinese herbalist diagnosed her condition as an excessively Cold state resulting from her predominantly vegetable diet. He made her a soup of eel, an energy food, and Angelica Sinensis 當歸, a warming and tonifying Blood herb often used for gynecologic maladies. After this dietary treatment, her excessive bleeding stopped. While eel is on the list of high-energy foods, it is less often used than frogs' legs because of its high cholesterol content.

Postmenopausal women in their sixth decade, when they are no longer having hot flashes, sometimes ingest large quantities of bean curd (tofu) or soymilk for the phytoestrogen content. If overdone, this can be harmful. At that time of life, the kidney Yang energy is often low. If taken in large quantities, soy and bean curds, which are considered cool, need to be counterbalanced with warming foods.

Westerners have a one-sided view of foods. They consider consuming green tea, leafy green vegetables, and a variety of fruits as completely virtuous because they contain phytonutrients that prevent cancer by way of their anti-inflammatory effects. Many are antioxidants. Others, like flavanoids, also stimulate the COX-1 pathway to prevent inflammation (Perricone 2004, 48). Let us not forget, though, that there is a complex Yin-Yang relationship between COX-1 and COX-2 pathways (see chapter 5). Many of these foods containing the highly touted cancer-preventing phytonutrients fall into the Cold category in the Eastern paradigm. Excessive use of them can lead to an imbalance. If the patient's constitution is thrown into a Cold state, adverse consequences might ensue. Inflammation is a Yang function. An excessively Cold condition can mean that the Yang energy necessary for immune function is suboptimal.

Yin-Promoting 養陰 Foods

In winter, when the cold weather dries the skin and mucous membranes, Chinese families often make soups with various squashes, dates, and figs. Slow, prolonged cooking with these ingredients and some pork will move vegetables in the cool category, such as bok choy or watercress, into a neutral position (neither hot nor cold). These soups are considered lubricating or tonifying to Yin because they help to moisten the mucous membranes.

The meat and shell of the turtle, a slow phlegmatic animal, is considered Yin. Turtle soup is believed to be therapeutic in Yin-deficient 陰虛 states, which include any condition where there is dryness. Flu, pneumonia, and radiation therapy all cause drying of a patient's mucous membranes. The Chinese practitioner would recommend turtle soup, considered a delicacy, to restore Yin in these patients. Other meats that promote Yin are abalone, rabbit, and wild duck (as opposed to farmed duck).

Foods that seem to be especially effective in moistening the lung 養肺陰 are loquats, cumquats, pears, and almonds, which are also frequently added to soups. These foods seem to not only nourish the Yin (enhance body fluid production) but also restore the normal consistency of mucous, which can become abnormally thick following a respiratory infection.

Dispersing Blood 散血 Foods

Some foods considered cold 涼 can also disperse blood 散血, or discourage blood from clotting. Such was my discovery with bitter melon 苦瓜. Nellie was a Chinese patient of mine in her eighties.

She suffered from chronic atrial fibrillation, a heart condition that put her at an increased risk for strokes. For stroke prevention, I prescribed coumadin to thin her blood. I adjusted her coumadin dosage by regularly monitoring her prothrombin time, which indicated how thin her blood was. After she had been on coumadin for quite a while, when the dosing requirement should have been stable, there were wide swings in her prothrombin time. Sometimes they were extremely high, indicating her blood was too thin. I would then have to tell Nellie to cut way down on her coumadin dosage.

Shortly before I retired, Nellie and her sister, also my patient, took me out to dinner. They asked me to pick something from the menu I liked, and I chose bitter melon sautéed with meat. Nellie commented that the dish was also one of her favorites, but she was afraid to eat much of it because every time she had bitter melon, she would receive my phone call informing her that her blood was too thin and that she had to reduce her coumadin dosage. I then realized that bitter melon, classified as a cool-cold vegetable, besides having antibacterial or antiviral functions, might also have anticlotting properties. I remember that when I was an adolescent, my mother advised me not to eat cool fruits like watermelon and bananas during my menses in order to avoid excessive bleeding. Perhaps the explanation is that these cool fruits also discourage clotting.

It is common in Chinese cooking to use ingredients that disperse blood 散血. Many of these foods are in the fungus family, such as black mushrooms 冬菇, cloud ears 雲耳, and wood ears 木耳. Years ago, I read in the *New England Journal of Medicine* about a case where researchers had to interrupt their study because of a puzzling development. The blood of the presumed normal subject, a Chinese researcher, intermittently had trouble clotting (Hammerschmidt 1980). The researchers discovered that the abnormality occurred on the days after the subject had eaten a dinner of Ma Paw Tofu 麻婆豆腐, which contained wood ears 木耳, a common fungus.

According to Chinese folk medicine, eating wood ear promotes longevity. This fungus most likely has antiplatelet properties, which help prevent strokes and heart attacks. We can think of it as comparable to taking one baby aspirin a day as so many older people in Western countries do.

In the 1950s, before the development of lipid-lowering drugs, my father would drink chrysanthemum 菊花 tea before having blood drawn to test his cholesterol level. He relied on the tea to keep his cholesterol down to an acceptable level. Chrysanthemum is categorized as a cool 凉 herb. TCM practitioners use it for treating eye diseases and lowering blood pressure. Chinese lay people traditionally drink it after a greasy meal because they believe it somehow neutralizes the grease. The properties of chrysanthemum might be explained in Western terms as lipid lowering and decreasing sympathetic activity.

Table 5 summarizes the TCM classification of some common foods.

For thousands of years, the Chinese have used this ancient system of food classifications to keep themselves well. My grandmother, who lived to be ninety-nine, saw a Western practitioner only twice in her lifetime, once for gallstones for which she refused surgery and once for a broken hip for which she did have surgery. She otherwise kept herself healthy with traditional Chinese ways. When she reached ninety, she said that she needed to decrease sweets because she was getting old. This was long before the low-carb rage and the discovery that high glycemic index foods are bad for cardiovascular health. When we consider the escalating cost of drugs, learning from these dietary teachings may serve us well in the areas of preventive medicine and cost containment.

Table 5. TCM Classification of Common Foods.

Toxic	Wet-*Hot*	Hot Qi	Warm-*Hot*	Neutral	Cool-*Cold*	Moisten Yin	Disperse Blood	Energy Meats
clam	beet	barbecued food	chili	apple	banana	abalone	bitter melon	beef
crab	cherry	chips	chocolate	apricot	cantaloupe	almonds	black mushroom	frogs' legs
duck	garlic	chocolate	cinnamon	avocado	carrots	cumquat	wood ear	lamb
lobster	mango	fried food	curry	chicken	celery	dates		venison
shrimp	orange	nuts	ginger	corn	cilantro	figs		
turkey	shallots	hot spices	jalapeno	fish	grapefruit	loquat		
	strawberry		pepper	grapes	green beans	rabbit		
	turnip		red beans	kiwi	honeydew	turtle		
				peach	leafy greens	wild duck		
				plum	lemon			
				pork	mint			
				pomegranate	pears			
				potatoes	watermelon			
				prune	winter melons			
				yam				
				zucchini				

"Nature, time and patience are the three great physicians."

— CHINESE PROVERB

Chapter 12
Adapting TCM to a Contemporary Western Practice

The following is a recent e-mail from my friend Amy:

> I have had migraine/sinus headaches for a number of years. It is funny that they happen mostly on weekends, and I have tried several kinds of Chinese doctors such as herbal doctors, "chi-kung" massage/herbal doctors, and acupuncture/herbal doctors as well. Not much has helped until recently. I went back to the herbal doctor who treated me years ago (I did not get better then). He said my kidney is a bit weak, thus making my hormones imbalanced—I am not sure if this is the right term. Well, this time I am getting a bit better because my weekly headaches are not as severe as before. I asked the herbal doctor if I am close to menopause, but he answered not quite yet.
>
> If you ask me why I do not go to a doctor who practices Western medicine, the answer is I have been to my family doctor and all he prescribes for headaches are painkillers, with the dosages

getting higher. I have had an MRI and CAT scan done; nothing was wrong. That is why I turned to Chinese herbal doctors instead.

Amy's plight is common to many patients with conditions for which mainstream Western medicine lacks satisfactory answers. The MRI and CAT scans were not helpful in either defining her condition or directing her doctor toward effective treatment. Her doctor prescribed stronger and stronger analgesics, but Amy wanted a cure, not just temporary pain relief. Her only recourse was to seek alternative caregivers without involving her primary care physician. Not knowing which type of practitioner would meet her needs, she sought a series of them. When she found one practitioner who seemed to help her, she was unsure of what he meant when he told her that her "kidneys were weak," and there was no one to translate.

What began for me as a small family practice that additionally offered TCM in a sublet office space evolved into a busy practice. Patients like Amy were desperate for a Western physician sympathetic to and knowledgeable about alternative treatments. Although I could not subscribe to extreme deviations from allopathic medicine such as the Candida theory of disease or the environmental allergists' approach of totally isolating patients from their environment, I did offer reasonable alternatives. I still used allopathic remedies for the majority of patients. For treating hypertension, I found that drugs were easier than herbs to titrate, but I sometimes supplemented a drug regimen with antihypertensive herbs. Over the years, various herbal teas came in and out of favor for lowering cholesterol, but when I let my patients take them and monitored their blood cholesterols, I found most were ineffective in changing their lab measurements. My patients with advanced coronary artery disease still underwent bypass surgery. After surgery, I would maintain them on the usual aspirin and cholesterol-lowering drugs and also supplement the drugs with herbs that promote blood flow. My diabetics still received diabetes teaching and drugs, but I prescribed Spleen tonifying herbs and also mobilizing-blood herbs to help with all the complications that accompany their disease. For women with severe menopausal symptoms, I prescribed hormone replacement for short-term relief at modest doses and supplemented with herbs for lowering Deficiency Fire (see chapter 2).

The challenge I faced was how to find ways to adapt ancient TCM treatments to a busy modern practice. I continued to use standard Western diagnostic methods, and if I recognized conditions for which I felt a TCM approach would be preferable, I presented patients with options and informed them of the respective pros and cons of each treatment plan. I pointed out that TCM would require more commitment of time and expense. In the early 1990s, it was rare for insurance companies to cover such treatments. I began to discover what a difference there was between TCM and allopathic medicine in terms of their demand on a practitioner's time and energy. For acupuncture, the patient occupied one of my three treatment rooms for forty minutes. A steroid injection would have taken ten minutes at most. Clearly, my motive for continuing to use TCM was not profit-driven. I used it because I believed in its effectiveness and safety. I could write an allopathic prescription in a matter of seconds; if I used a TCM approach, I had to wait until the end of the day when I had the time to laboriously write a twelve- to fourteen-ingredient herbal prescription using Chinese script, which I would then mail to the patient. I really appreciated the advent of the fax machine, which eliminated a lot of mailing. Once, though, I dialed the wrong number and, much to their bewilderment, people working at a bank, instead of my patient, received the Chinese prescription.

As to the creed of mainstream medicine that steroids are the drugs of choice for joint injections, I had become an apostate. I had seen too many adverse effects and therefore looked for alternatives. A podiatrist, who practiced sports medicine using a complementary approach, told me he used a homeopathic solution for injecting soft tissue (Subotnick 1991, 199). When I began using it for injecting soft tissue inflammation, I was impressed with the results, and it became my injectable solution of choice. With steroids, after the local anesthetic wears off, the patient has an intensification of pain for the first one or two days before relief finally sets in. This did not occur with the homeopathic injection.

Another colleague, a physician acupuncturist, said that he succeeded in treating allergic rhinitis by using a vitamin B12 injection at acupuncture points around the nose. I adopted his technique. My results were unexpected and inexplicable. The best responders to this treatment were young males. For females and older men, the treatment had no effect. Every spring, a number of my younger male patients would come in for their injection into the Bitong acupuncture point for their hay fever, and they would be asymptomatic for the season.

I had discovered an herbalist who concentrated herbal formulas into tinctures. One of his tinctures was for colds and the flu. If taken early, at the first warning sign of the flu, when there was just a slight sore throat, it would stop the progression to full-blown symptoms. This led to another tradition among my patients. In the fall, about the time I began giving flu shots, mothers would come in to get a supply of the tincture to protect their families against the onslaught of the flu.

For patients who had flu that had progressed beyond the initial sore throat, I wrote three standardized prescriptions for different stages of the flu, and would merely copy the appropriate one for each patient. I individualized by adding a few herbs here and there.

Using TCM for a Cancer Patient

I continued to adhere to the standard of practice of the allopathic medical community. Because cancer patients were usually under the care of an oncologist who rarely approved of alternative treatments, I chose not to assume TCM care for those patients. I routinely referred them to Dr. Lai. An exception was Mrs. O. She had chosen me as her primary care physician through her HMO. Her options for health-care providers were limited to the HMO panel. Mrs. O. had a rare cancer of the muscle that had spread to her lungs. It was inoperable, and neither radiation nor chemotherapy was considered effective. In view of these circumstances, her oncologist had no objection to alternative treatments. I ventured to treat Mrs. O. with Chinese herbs using the principle of balancing cleansing herbs to fight the cancer and immune boosting herbs to help her body fight the disease. In her eighties, Mrs. O. remained functional with a good quality of life for her remaining two and a half years. She was an artist and continued to paint, and she was able to take public transportation everywhere.

Each winter, Mrs. O. suffered a bout of respiratory infection. Each time she responded well to an old and inexpensive antibiotic, ampicillin. I knew that with her lung metastases, her demise would most likely be from respiratory problems. I shared my plans for terminal care with her daughter. When the end was near, I would admit her mother not to the acute hospital but to a facility with a hospice-like setting, where she could receive oxygen and an intravenous morphine drip. Mrs. O.'s last days were as I had anticipated. Her daughter sat by her bedside, playing Mrs. O.'s favorite music on a cassette recorder, and in a matter of days, Mrs. O. passed on very peacefully.

Using TCM to Treat Avascular Necrosis of the Hip

Martha, in her late thirties, developed Stevens-Johnson syndrome, a rare allergic-type reaction, from taking an antiseizure drug. She became severely ill with a skin rash, mouth sores, and a high fever. She was hospitalized and treated with high doses of steroids. Two months after her discharge from the hospital, Martha told me she had pain in one hip. A dreaded complication of steroid therapy is avascular necrosis of the hip where the blood supply to the head of the femur (hipbone) becomes inadequate, and the bone disintegrates. I suspected this to be what was wrong, and my diagnosis was confirmed with a bone scan and MRI.

The orthopedist I consulted told me that sometimes even a very small dose of a steroid could cause avascular necrosis. At Martha's young age, he did not advise a total hip replacement, which usually requires revisions about every ten years. He told me about an operation that involves making tiny holes in the head of the femur to stimulate circulation to this part of the bone, but it was not always successful. The Western options did not sound favorable. I consulted Dr. Lai to see if there were any effective TCM therapies. He advised me to use an herb formula often used for arthritis to increase circulation to the bone. After Martha had been on the formula for four months, the orthopedist repeated the MRI, and it showed some healing of the hip bone. When I retired eight years later, Martha still had not required surgery.

TCM's Role in Cost Containment

During my later practice, something new in health care became increasingly prevalent: the Health Maintenance Organization (HMO) system. The concept is that health-care providers, including doctors, are paid only a flat fee up front whether the patient requires a lot of care or only a little. This puts the onus on the doctor to keep the patient as healthy as possible. The common goal of maintaining health to contain cost is sound. But I found the HMO's method of rules and regulations often self-defeating. The ultimate arbiter of how a patient was managed was no longer the patient's physician but some clerk with no medical background, a clerk who made life and death decisions by using an algorithm from an inert database. It seemed ironic that when I phoned to request approval of a test or treatment, the clerk on the other end of the phone would ask, "How do you spell that diagnosis?"

When I worked under a single HMO system, the rule was that every doctor was allotted enough time to see and treat six patients an hour, which meant ten minutes per patient, regardless of the complexity of the problem. I recall seeing a patient who had already made four visits without having his problem solved. On his fifth visit, I spent an extra five minutes to obtain a more detailed history, and, because of that effort, I was able to solve his problem. Yet I was criticized for spending more than the allotted time. The critics failed to compute the time spent on the patient's four previous unfruitful visits.

In about the mid-1990s, some HMOs began covering acupuncture services. The medical director of the group I was affiliated with asked if I could help create guidelines for the use of acupuncture. I read the proposed guidelines, which stated, "Acupuncture is covered when all other forms of conventional therapy have been tried and failed." What a paradox, I thought. HMO's main goal is cost-effective care. If all other therapies had to be tried before the potentially effective one, acupuncture, is contemplated, the cost of care will escalate rather than being contained. I suggested deleting that guideline and replacing it with a list of conditions for which I knew acupuncture to be effective.

Focusing on cost containment, modern health delivery systems need to realize that time plays an important role in determining how patient care evolves. In earlier days, a common scenario was that when a patient called the doctor at night, the doctor would say, "Take two aspirins and call me in the morning." There is more wisdom to this advice than first appears. If the body is given a chance, many conditions spontaneously resolve. For instance, when a patient first has a cough without fever, and his physical examination shows his lungs to be clear, a doctor will most likely wait a week or ten days to see if the symptoms resolve before launching into a costly workup. Often, if the cause of the symptoms is a common viral respiratory infection, the patient will get better on his or her own. If the symptoms persist, then the wheels of costly workup begin to roll, including X-rays, CT scans, and bronchoscopy. Depending on the condition, sometimes the test results are helpful but sometimes they are not.

A common example of how the cost of working up a persistent problem escalates can be seen with patients who suffer from soft tissue inflammation such as tendonitis and cervical or lumbar discitis. If the patient can be treated early with acupuncture and the symptoms resolve, no further workup is necessary. On the other hand, if initial treatment using Western modalities proves ineffective, the inevitable next step is costly imaging, such as an MRI. Often the MRI gives no definitive answers. I have repeatedly seen patients who have already spent thousands of dollars on tests that failed to point the way to definitive treatment before finally coming for acupuncture, which finally helped them.

The following three cases are examples of how using TCM resulted in considerable medical cost savings.

A Case of Cervical Disc Disease

Brenda, a patient in her mid-fifties, complained of one-sided neck pain radiating down the arm on the same side. I suspected she had a degenerative cervical disc, partially herniating and pinching the nerve to her arm. I planned to confirm my diagnosis with an X-ray and then treat with acupuncture. I told Brenda to go downstairs to the X-ray department. About twenty minutes later, Brenda returned saying the line in the X-ray department was very long and she would rather get the treatment first. I proceeded to acupuncture her for cervical disc disease. After the treatment, Brenda arose from the table. "I don't need to go for the X-ray; my neck already feels much better," she told me. I then gave Brenda a series of six treatments at weekly intervals, and she had no recurrences of her symptoms.

A Case of PMS and Infertility

Terry, in her late thirties, came to see me for acupuncture to treat severe PMS. Once, during that time of the month, her mind was so clouded that she drove into a parked car. She also had severe menstrual cramps. Suspecting she might have endometriosis, a condition that can involve severe menstrual pain, I asked if she had received a gynecology workup. She said she was considering it but wanted to try acupuncture first. After ten sessions, she improved greatly. She felt good before her periods, and they were no longer painful. Terry then told me that she had been married for four years and had never conceived despite not using contraception. I again asked if she had received a Western workup, and she again said she preferred to try acupuncture first. I continued acupuncturing her, and four months later, Terry became pregnant and later gave birth to a beautiful baby girl. When you consider the cost of today's high-tech fertility treatments, acupuncture certainly is a viable option.

A Case of Obstructive Pulmonary Disease

My friend Irene was diagnosed with lung cancer twice. She was a nonsmoker who had no previous lung problems. The first time, she had surgery and two lobes of her right lung were removed. She was fine until two years later, when another cancer developed in her left lung. For that, the chest surgeon removed a wedge of lung tissue. Less than a week after she was discharged, she became extremely short of breath and was readmitted to the hospital with the complication of an empyema (an infection between the two layers of membranes covering her lung). The surgeon inserted a tube to drain the pus. After the procedure, her shortness of breath was no better. Because the infection was not responding to antibiotics, she underwent another operation called decortication, to remove the infected lung membrane. Her shortness of breath continued. She could not cough up her thick sputum. Her lung specialist felt that she had developed obstructive pulmonary disease after her surgeries, but he faced a dilemma. He was already treating with around-the-clock inhaled beta agonists to dilate her bronchial tubes without much improvement. With her complicated infection, he feared that using steroids for bronchodilation might weaken her ability to fight infection. When I visited her, Irene was barely able to walk ten feet around the hospital ward without being winded. She had already spent a month in the hospital. She reluctantly agreed to take the herbs I offered to brew for her after I promised her it would not taste too awful. The formula was one that I had often used for post-flu bronchitis. Because the prescription did not contain bitter tasting cold-cleansing herbs, the concoction was palatable. After two doses, she was able to walk around the hospital ward, and in less than a week, she was able to go home. She continued herbal therapy for three months. She has since felt well enough to fly to Virginia to babysit her granddaughter and fly to Hawaii to see her son. She was even able to participate in an antiwar march.

If anyone asks me whether TCM is cost effective, my answer would be, "If used appropriately, a resounding yes!" When subjected to HMO scrutiny, my practice was at the high end for cost-effectiveness. I used acupuncture in about 20 percent of my practice. I probably ordered fewer expensive imaging tests than any other physician with a comparable practice. I did not need to when I saw my patients responding to the TCM approach.

In later years, it was gratifying to see more of my medical colleagues becoming interested in what I was doing. Even the chiefs of family practice, internal medicine, and orthopedics at my hospital referred patients with musculoskeletal soft tissue disorders to me for acupuncture treatment. I was invited to speak both to medical colleagues and to the lay public about TCM. I was delighted at the opportunity to inform both doctors and patients about what options were available and the conditions for which I found TCM effective. There seemed to be a general awakening to the vision I had so distantly seen long ago as a third-year medical student. Indeed, TCM has a role in modern times.

Chapter 13

A Comparison of the Western and Eastern Paradigms

I n the 1990s, as I accepted more invitations to lecture on Eastern medicine, a field that was receiving ever-increasing attention, I tried to define some of the differences between the Eastern and Western paradigms.

Before I fully understood TCM, I had maintained a monolithic view: what was taught in medical school was the only medical paradigm. Now I realize that Western medicine is actually a product of Cartesian philosophy. In college, philosophy was not one of my favorite subjects. It is only recently that I have come to understand what a profound effect philosophy has had on the development of society in general and on medicine in particular. Just as Taoism shaped the course of Eastern medicine, Descartes, the sixteenth-century philosopher who said, "I think, therefore I am," shaped the course of Western medicine.

Mechanistic vs. Organic

One day, I described to Dr. Lai how a patient with infertility was worked up by Western practitioners: first a laparoscopy was performed to view the status of her reproductive organs, then came laser lysis of adhesions from endometriosis, and then came the hysterosalpingogram to check if her tubes were open. He mused, "These Americans treat the female reproductive tract like a car—clean and tune the engine, check out the hoses—and they expect it to function." This mechanistic approach can be understood if we recognize that it comes from Cartesian philosophy.

Descartes likened the human being to two clocks: one is the body and the other, the mind, each running independently of the other and of its surroundings. The parts of the clock are uniform for all individuals. When a malfunction occurs, you take the clock apart, find and fix the broken part, and function is restored (Osborne 1992, 70–75). The Western tradition of analysis came from this concept.

Cartesian philosophy also accounts for the prevailing Western notion that if the patient's illness cannot be explained with available tests on the body, then it must, by default, be in the patient's mind and not worthy of any further investigation or attention. Exploration of the mind-body connection is a recent Western medical trend. We are regarding this connection as if it were a newly discovered concept. It is novel to us only because we have forgotten that before Descartes, the mind and body were not separated.

Early in my integrated practice, a man from somewhere in the Midwest phoned to seek my help as an acupuncturist. He told me he was desperate to get relief, even if he had to fly west to see me. His problem began after a hernia operation that was complicated postoperatively by an infection in his testicle. The surgeon must have thought that if the testicle hurt so much, he could solve the problem by removing it. After the testicle was removed, the patient suffered even more from agonizing phantom pain. Still new to practicing acupuncture, I was unsure if acupuncture could help him and advised him against making the long journey to see me. Later, he called back to tell me he had obtained relief from an antidepressant drug. We now know antidepressants work for pain relief via their action on pain pathways in the nervous system independent of their antidepressant effects. This man's story was a poignant reminder to me of the fallacy of viewing the human organism as a machine. Years ago my family doctor explained PMS to me as "the cry of the dying ovum." I believe today's widespread pursuit of complementary care represents the Western patient's cry: "I am not a machine."

In Chinese landscape painting, people are depicted as a tiny portion of the whole landscape. This reflects the Eastern world-view that man is but a tiny part of the cosmos. An extension of this Eastern concept is that the human organism itself is a microcosm, where the sum of all parts, including the mind and body, are inter-related, and cannot be separated from the whole. Disease can occur when there is a disruption of the normal harmony between man and the cosmos. It can also occur when, within the microcosm of man himself, there is a disruption in the homeostatic mechanisms responsible for maintaining normalcy. The Eastern view takes into account the external and internal, past and present, and aims not only to treat the body's external invaders but also to restore the patient's balance.

Focusing on the Present vs. Connecting the Present to the Past

Years ago, a patient in his early forties came to see me seeking acupuncture for pain in his right groin. His past medical history included a testicular cancer on that side, which was removed suc-cessfully when he was in his twenties. At the time, still inexperi-enced, I intuitively asked if there could be a relationship between the past surgery and the present pain. He rejected that idea, insist-ing that the surgery was long ago, the wound had healed, and the whole thing was only past history. He proceeded to ask how many cases of this type I had treated. "Not many," I told him. With his Western mindset, he was intent on finding an acupuncturist who specialized or had a lot of experience treating groin pain. Still accustomed to the Western way of thinking, I told him I knew of no one and probably could not help him. In retrospect, with my added years of experience, I think there was a relationship between his past surgery and his pain. If I had resisted the pull of his Western way of thinking and hung on to my original conviction, I probably could have helped him.

I once attended a conference on acupuncture treatment of back pain. To demonstrate her technique, the lecturer asked for volunteers from the audience who had back problems. A woman in her forties stood up as a willing subject. She said she was not a back pain sufferer now, but anticipated problems in the future. She gave the following explanation. In her family, the men carried a genetic defect that caused them to lose kidney function at a young age. The women in the family were free from this genetically transmitted disease and donated their kidneys to the men. Usually about twenty years after the women donated their kidneys, they developed back problems, and most of them had to undergo lumbar laminectomies. She had recently donated her kidney to a cousin. She wanted treatments to prevent the lower back problems the other kidney donors in her family had developed. This sounded fascinating. I went up to talk to her after the lecture and asked if the transplant surgeons knew about this complication of the kidney donors. She answered that because the complication was so remote from the time of surgery, the surgeons were not aware of it.

This story made me realize how shortsighted we tend to be. I began to think of cases I had treated in the past. There was the physician who had a childhood leg injury. It was not until two decades later that she developed back and leg pain, and I treated her with acupuncture. There was the elderly patient who had undergone hip replacement. Her course was complicated by postoperative bleeding, and she required reoperation. She saw me for persistent hip pain for which no apparent cause could be found. Her surgeon told her the X-rays and MRIs had shown a successful hip replacement. I found the muscles around her hip area were tense, and when I loosened them using acupuncture, her pain was relieved.

These cases seemed to have a common theme. After a procedure or trauma, the body's muscles guard the area by tightening around it, leading to problems years later. In the case of the kidney donors, when the muscles of the back on the operated side tightened, they gradually caused a curvature in the spine. With years of this abnormal pull, the disc space on that side became narrowed, resulting in lumbar disc disease. Western medicine needs to recognize that the past does influence the present.

Reductionism vs. Integration

If we begin with the premise that the body is a clock, logic dictates that when it malfunctions, we must take it apart in order to locate the problem. The Cartesian tradition is analytical, reducing things to the smallest common denominator in search of the cause for malfunctions. The penultimate example is the mapping of the human genome. This approach makes specificity paramount. Treatment is targeted for a specific cause. To treat a serious bacterial infection, for example, Western medicine takes a specimen such as blood or sputum, cultures it to identify the offending microorganism, and runs further tests to determine which antimicrobials are the most effective in killing the microorganism.

The perceived need for specificity permeates Western thinking among both doctors and patients. Sometimes it is carried to extremes. The assumption is that until the diagnosis is completely clarified with minute testing, treatment cannot be determined. When patients do not improve, they often ask for more tests "to find out what's wrong with me." Even then, the most sophisticated tests may not shed any further light on their problems. This not only drives up the cost of health care, it delays needed treatment.

One patient of mine had been in an automobile accident in which he sustained a back injury. He had undergone surgery for lumbar disc herniation. After the surgery, he continued to have residual pain in his back, radiating down his leg in the typical sciatic nerve distribution. He also complained of pain at the tip of his penis. Looking at my neuroanatomy book, I noted that the distribution of his penile pain was precisely the area supplied by the S2 nerve root. I told him his pain was most likely from the nerve root to his penis having been injured in the accident. Not satisfied with that explanation, he sought out a urologist who proceeded to perform a cystoscopy to look inside his urethra and bladder. The urologist found no pathology in the urinary tract, but the patient suffered the complication of a bladder infection after the procedure. When I later asked him why he had gone through all that suffering for naught, he answered, "I just wanted to be sure of what was wrong with me."

Cartesian reductionism also accounts for the trend toward specialization, and even sub-specialization, in medicine. When specialist care becomes the initial step, we sometimes lose sight of the forest for the trees. Before coming to see me for primary care, a patient went to multiple eye specialists for discomfort in her eyes. The specialists repeatedly told her there was nothing wrong with her eyes. When I saw her, I discovered that an overactive thyroid gland was causing her symptoms. Eye discomfort with bulging is a common accompaniment of Grave's Disease. Western patients share a common misconception that if they can only find a super-specialist to deal with the body part giving them symptoms, their problems will be solved. Unfortunately, the human organism, contrary to Descartes' teaching, is not always so simple as the sum of its parts.

Anne was fourteen years old when she began having lower abdominal pain, back pain, and severe constipation. Through an HMO system, she had seen a pediatrician and an emergency room physician. For her back pain, a back X-ray was ordered. For her constipation, a dietary consultation was ordered. The back X-ray showed scoliosis. She was then sent to a back specialist who determined that her back pain was not from a disease of the back. The diet recommended did not help her constipation. By the time she came to see me, the patient and her parents were very frustrated. Since she had constipation, I thought the most basic examination was in order. As soon as I performed the rectal exam, I found a large pelvic mass. I referred her to a gynecologist. After performing an examination under anesthesia, the gynecologist found that Anne had an abnormal reproductive tract, causing obstruction to normal flow of menstrual blood. The mass I felt on rectal exam was actually the accumulation of blood in her vagina. All her symptoms came from it. Pressure from this mass caused pain in the lower abdomen and back. Pressure on the rectum from it accounted for her constipation. The reason Anne's case took so long to unravel was that her previous physicians, rather than listening to her story and performing a basic physical examination, had been distracted with specialized tests.

TCM treatment does not depend on a specific diagnosis. Chinese medicine therefore does not require extensive testing. It uses an integrative approach. To diagnose, TCM practitioners just need to determine which system is out of balance. Multiple herbs with similar actions are prescribed to barrage the offending "evil," along with herbs to rebalance the host's ability to fight disease. Acupuncture directs blood flow to the area that is diseased and helps the body to take over and normalize itself.

Focusing on Disease vs. Disease and Host

The Western premise that the body is like a machine implies that the body has no inherent ability to repair itself and therefore requires a mechanic to repair it. Consequently, Western medicine focuses on conquering disease rather than on the host's ability to fight disease. At times, this approach can lead to some measure of harm because the battleground is the body itself. To some degree, treatment to attack the invader can also undermine the host's well-being. To address this, Western medicine targets the disease with increasing specificity to minimize harm to the host. The development of monoclonal antibodies, which attack cancer cells specifically and leave all other cells alone, is an example.

Eastern treatment uses a two-pronged approach, directing attention not only at the causative invader but also at strengthening the host. My friend Frances, a missionary in China, e-mailed me about her medical problem. She was having bladder infections one after another despite multiple courses of antibiotic treatments, including one prolonged course. It seemed as soon as she was off antibiotics, she would suffer another bout of bladder infection. After three months, the strain of bacteria causing her infection was getting resistant to almost all antibiotics. Her doctors, at an impasse, were planning to study her immune system. The test results later turned out to be normal. She noticed that the beginning of her symptoms seemed to have coincided with the discontinuation of estrogen replacement hormones, a decision prompted by recent warnings about estrogen replacement therapy being linked to cancer. Frances told me that twenty years ago, when she was in her forties, she developed uterine fibroids for which she underwent surgery. About a year after her surgery, she had severe pain on her right side, and she underwent a second operation. Her surgeons found that she had a pelvic infection, a complication of the first surgery. They also found so much scarring and abscess formation around the ovaries that they had to remove them. She was then put on estrogen replacement until very recently. Using my TCM background, I reasoned that with all the complications of her surgery, her pelvic organs, including the bladder, had undergone scarring, and the blood supply to these organs was inadequate. The twenty years of estrogen replacement was what maintained her normal bladder immunity. When that was discontinued, her bladder's ability to fight bacterial infection was compromised. I advised her to use a topical estrogen cream and e-mailed a prescription of herbs that tonify the Kidney, restore Yin to the pelvic mucous membranes, and promote circulation to the pelvic area. After about three weeks on this regimen, her bladder infections no longer recurred. Whereas the Western approach focused mainly on her bladder infection, the Eastern approach focused on the patient.

Structural vs. Functional

Since Western medicine likens the body to a clock, the natural corollary is that you either take it apart to fix it or somehow peer inside to find the malfunctioning part. We have therefore devised methods of looking into any and every orifice possible, from gastroesophagoscopy, to colonoscopy, and now to ductoscopy (looking inside the milk ducts of the breast). The goal of these diagnostic procedures is to find a structural abnormality that Western science can treat. In a common scenario, the patient does not feel well and sees the allopathic doctor. When the physical examination shows no abnormalities, tests are ordered. If the complaint is gastrointestinal distress, for example, the tests will probably include looking into either the upper or lower GI tract or both. A few days later, the physician informs the patient of the good news. "All your tests are normal." The patient then wonders, "If all my tests are normal, what is wrong with me?" The patient may not recognize that the tests are for structure, not function.

The absence of structural abnormalities does not exclude functional problems. In this example, nerves to the intestines may not be working optimally for normal synchronous motion. Actually, the term "functional" carries a definite connotation. To the mind of a Western practitioner, "functional" means the problem is not serious; it does not require much attention; it is most likely just in the patient's mind, and it can be dismissed. Deeper in the physician's mind is the knowledge that Western medicine does not offer many good treatment options for functional conditions. Structural problems are those that we excel in treating. Before studying TCM, I also held this view.

One patient's story is a sad caricature of the attitude I used to share with so many Western colleagues. Herman was a middle-aged man who had led a life sheltered from the medical system. One day he went to the local hospital emergency room for chest pain. He was quickly admitted to the coronary care unit. He described with bewilderment the way he was treated. "In one instant, the hospital staff treated me with such care, as if I were a delicate rose. They did not allow me to pick up even the lightest of objects. In the next instant, when the tests all came back normal, ruling out a heart attack, they could not push me out their door fast enough." Testing had moved Herman's chest pain from the structural to the functional bin. In a flash, Herman, once the center of attention, became a nonentity in his caregivers' eyes. If mainstream practitioners ever wonder why disenchanted patients are flocking to complementary practitioners, they should examine themselves.

Taoism influenced Eastern medicine to shun invasion of the body. While Eastern practitioners have fewer solutions for structural abnormalities, which represent a more advanced stage of disease, they do offer viable solutions for functional abnormalities. TCM directs treatment at encouraging the body to regain normal function.

Replace vs. Restore

Western medicine fixes malfunctioning parts by replacing them. When someone has degenerative arthritis, Western practitioners wait until the joint is completely destroyed and then replace it. When blood vessels are occluded, such as in coronary heart disease, we replace them with normal blood vessels from other parts of the body. When a larger vessel such as the aorta is involved, we replace it with an artificial vessel. Western medicine addresses early disease with "watchful waiting."

Eastern medicine uses a different approach. It aims to restore malfunctioning parts so that they will function longer. Acupuncture tends to improve circulation to the joint and surrounding muscles, forestalling further degeneration in the joint. For vascular occlusive disease, TCM practitioners can use herbs that discourage arteriosclerotic plaque formation.

I once saw a Public Broadcasting television program about the remarkable Egyptian obelisks (Pharaoh's Obelisk 1994). The modern project was to figure out how the early Egyptians were able to raise these magnificent tall structures to the upright position. A British engineer tried to devise a method simulating the resources available at that time. The obelisk was hoisted on a large crane and tied with ropes. Two hundred men, at a prescribed distance, were assigned to pull the ropes. As they pulled, the obelisk would begin to slide off its moorings. The task was finally abandoned because of the unnecessary danger to the men. But an American sculptor in the group was not willing to give up so easily. He used a different approach. By displacing the sand underneath the obelisk, he used the obelisk's own weight to shift and pivot itself to an upright position. I think this is a good analogy for comparing Western and Eastern medicine. Western medicine uses powerful external force to effect change, but it is accompanied by some risk. Eastern medicine leverages existing internal forces to achieve the same result with less risk.

"To everything there is a season, and a time for every purpose under the heaven."

— ECCLESIASTES 3:1

Chapter 14

The Yin and Yang of Integration

A ttitudes toward Eastern medicine often border on one of two
extremes. Some people feel complementary care cannot be
trusted because it lacks any scientific proof. Actually, science itself
stems from a belief system originating from Descartes with its own
set of biases. The Nobel Prize laureate in medicine, Paul Nurse,
said that science is tentative knowledge (2004). The apostle Paul
said, "Now I know in part." Our science textbooks constantly need
updating because we know only "in part." The West can learn from
the East to respect the whole.

The other attitude is at the opposite extreme. Some people
who have experienced unsatisfactory outcomes using the Western
approach have totally abandoned Western medicine. That is like
throwing the baby out with the bathwater. When I visited the
exhibit on Chinese astronomy at the Oakland Space and Science
Center, I saw the very cumbersome way the Chinese in antiquity
told time with a water clock as big as a refrigerator. While we are
still using the ancient Chinese astronomers' method to measure
longitude and latitude, I doubt if anyone would want to revert
to telling time with a water clock. What we need to do is pick

and choose what we want to retain from antiquity. The ancient Eastern approach and the modern Western approach both have their strengths and limitations. If we recognize what they are, we can truly use both disciplines in a complementary way and get the best of both worlds.

The advances made in Western medicine are second to none. Methods of imaging such as CT and MRI scanning, laparoscopic surgery, angioplasty, joint replacement, transplant surgery, fetal surgery, gene research, vaccine development, and genomics are just some that come to mind. The benefits they bring cannot be ignored. There are times, however, when Western medicine has limitations. Ideally, this is when TCM should be considered.

When to Use Eastern Medicine

There is a story of a patient suffering from the common cold. She saw her doctor, who prescribed some pills. She returned two days later to say she had developed a cough and was not any better. He then prescribed some cough syrup. Two days later, she returned to say she was still no better. He then advised her to take a warm bath, open the window wide, and stand in front of it. She said, "But if I do that, I'll catch pneumonia." "Well," he replied, "that's something I can treat."

For certain conditions, the Western approach is just not effective. A recent research study showed that the most common formula prescribed for nighttime cough in children was no better than a placebo (Paul 2004; Yoder, et al. 2006). From my experience as a third-year medical student suffering from a nagging cough, I can attest to that fact. We should consider that the Chinese herbal pharmacopoeia is replete with effective remedies for coughs.

Vertigo, the type of dizziness typified by a feeling of spinning, can have two causes. One is a problem with the inner ear or labyrinth where the center of balance is. The other cause is a decrease in blood flow to the brain, a possible warning sign of an impending stroke. Usually, the Western treatment for the labyrinthine problem is a motion sickness pill such as meclizine, which is not very effective. The treatment for the second, more serious problem, is aspirin or, if the patient is already on aspirin, an antiplatelet medication. In both cases, TCM can be of benefit, using herbs that improve circulation to the head such as Rhizoma et Radix Ligustici Sinensis 藁本 and Rhizoma Gastrodiae Elatae 天麻. For the labyrinthine problem, herbs alone often resolve the problem. For the poor cerebral circulation, herbs that improve circulation to the head can be used as adjunctive treatment. A certain portion of the population is allergic to aspirin; another portion experiences serious GI bleeding from aspirin, and another does not respond to aspirin (Cavallari, et al. 2006). For those patients, mobilizing-blood herbs can be considered in lieu of aspirin.

For kidney stones, the conservative Western approach is to have the patient increase fluid intake in hopes of flushing the stone through the ureter, the conduit that transports urine from the kidney to the bladder. The ureter is a tube whose walls are made of smooth muscle. It is the narrowest part of the entire urinary tract, and it is where most stones become impacted on their way to the bladder. The intense pain accompanying kidney stones is from the smooth muscle wall of the ureter reflexively contracting in an effort to move the stone down to the bladder. Once a stone passes through the ureter, it will easily be excreted in the urine. If the conservative approach fails, Western medicine resorts to invasive measures. One approach is to pulverize the stone using sound waves. Another is to extract the stone surgically. Both of these procedures carry risks. Here, again, we could consider using Chinese herbs such as Achyranthis Bidentatae 牛膝 that dilate the ureter by relaxing its smooth muscle wall in combination with herbs that are diuretic such as Caulis Mutong 木通. These herbs can be used as adjuncts to the conservative approach.

A patient for whom I prescribed herbs to facilitate passage of his kidney stone told me that after taking the herbal concoction, in addition to passing his stone, he felt, for the first time in his life, that his usually cold hands had become warm. The smooth-muscle-relaxing herb component of his prescription dilated not only his ureter but also his blood vessels. There is a condition called Raynaud's phenomenon in which the blood vessels to the hands and feet constrict and the extremities can become uncomfortably cold. Western practitioners often prescribe vasodilating drugs such as nifedipine for it. Mobilizing Qi and Blood herbs that dilate blood vessels can also be effective (see chapters 3 and 9).

Another factor to consider when choosing one treatment over another is the risk/benefit ratio. Every treatment involves some risk. For life-threatening diseases, significant risk could be deemed justifiable. Yet drugs with serious side effects are often used for conditions that pose no imminent danger. This is when we should be cognizant of alternatives.

For simple strains, sprains, and tendonitis, accepted Western treatment is nonsteroidal anti-inflammatory drugs (NSAIDs). The first generation of NSAIDs can cause gastritis with GI bleeding and sometimes cause kidney failure. Short-term use to control symptoms might be justifiable, but for chronic use, the benefit does not warrant the risk. We thought the newer generation of NSAIDs called the COX-2 inhibitors would be the solution to the GI bleeding problem, but now we are discovering that they carry a new, unforeseen risk of increasing heart attacks and strokes among some users (see chapter 5). Many conditions for which NSAIDs are being prescribed respond well to herbal therapy and acupuncture.

It is appalling to find advertisements promoting NSAIDs to treat such benign conditions as the common cold. There is a case in which a child was given ibuprofen for a sore throat and developed Stevens-Johnson syndrome, a rare allergic reaction, which ultimately resulted in blindness. Chicken soup, herbs, or homeopathic remedies could have been used without such dreadful consequences.

Recently, higher doses of common painkillers such as acetaminophen and NSAIDs have been linked with hypertension in women (Dedier, et al. 2002). Now, more than ever; alternatives to drugs for treating pain should be considered.

Vasoconstricting drugs, such as phenylephrine, are known to cause hypertension, which can lead to strokes. Many drugs for nasal decongestion contain vasoconstrictors. The risk of a stroke is not commensurate with the benefit of nasal decongestion. Numerous herbs are equally effective and do not cause vasoconstriction.

Many diet pills also contain drugs that are vasoconstrictors. A common component is ephedrine. I used ephedrine as an anesthesiologist to help raise an excessively low blood pressure. Both TCM and Western practitioners have used ephedrine effectively for relieving bronchospasm in asthma and bronchitis. But its use for weight control is not appropriate. There has never been a drug proven to achieve sustained weight loss. Many have serious side effects, and using them is not justifiable. Herbal remedies that work on tonifying Spleen can offer a safer alternative.

In addition to the inherent risk with any surgery coupled with anesthesia, another problem with surgical procedures is scarring. Many patients have recurrences of their pain years after back surgery. Usually, they undergo repeat spine imaging. The common explanation for their pain is arachnoiditis (scarring of the membranes around the spinal cord). I saw a patient who had surgery for carpal tunnel syndrome with scarring that caused symptoms worse than that of her original problem. In such cases, acupuncture could have been a better first option.

For some common disorders, Eastern treatments are simpler and far less expensive. The West treats enuresis (bedwetting) with antidiuretic hormones and elaborate alarm systems to induce a conditioned response from the child with this problem. The Eastern treatment is simpler. It involves adding astringent herbs like Ootheca Mantidis 桑螵蛸 to a prescription that tonifies the Kidney. For difficulties with lactation, the West encourages the patient to drink fluids. In addition to fluids, the East offers herbs like Fructus Hordei Vulgaris Germanatus 麥芽 and Fructus Oryzae

Germinatus 谷芽 in a formula along with herbs to tonify the Blood, Yin, and Kidney Qi. For women's health issues such as premenstrual syndrome, irregular bleeding, menopausal symptoms, and infertility, Western methods of treatment are not all ideal. The Western treatment of PMS is not effective. Hormones for irregular bleeding and menopausal symptoms carry inherent risks. Infertility treatments are enormously expensive and not always successful. Eastern methods for these problems involve little risk, are often effective, and involve much lower cost.

When Not to Use Eastern Medicine

A balanced discussion of Eastern treatments must also include words of caution about their use. Some ancient remedies have withstood the test of time even though they were based on incorrect premises. For example, the TCM treatment for colds and the flu is used even today despite the fact that the treatment is based on the incorrect premise that colds and the flu are caused by the Cold evil.

But in some instances flawed premises have led to flawed treatments. A glaring example is diagnosing "Blood Stasis" as the cause of excessive uterine bleeding. It seems that when the ancients saw women with heavy menstrual bleeding passing clots (actually clots are an indication that the menstrual blood flow is brisker than normal), they assumed the clots were being formed in the uterine vessels and were responsible for obstructing normal menstrual flow (Wiseman 1995, 149). The TCM treatment is to mobilize Qi and Blood (see chapter 3). The intent of this treatment is to dissolve the offending clots in order to restore normal menstrual flow. Some of the herbs in this category act to disperse blood 散血. They act in a way similar to antiplatelet drugs like aspirin. They can have an anticoagulant effect and can worsen the bleeding. While there are various causes of excessive menstrual bleeding, excessive clotting is not one of them.

I once saw a patient who had pelvic pain. It was from an ectopic pregnancy. Before she came to me, she had consulted a Chinese herbalist who told her that the cause of the abnormal bleeding was "fire" in the reproductive organs. The diagnosis puzzled me, but I was glad she sought Western medical help in time. Delay would have resulted in severe and dangerous bleeding from her ectopic pregnancy. As I thought about the strange diagnosis the TCM practitioner gave this patient, "fire" in the reproductive organs, I remembered that one TCM teaching attributed early and heavy menstrual bleeding to Blood Heat (Wiseman 1996, 150). The ancients envisioned that the blood in the uterine vessels heated up to such a degree that it boiled over, leading to copious menstrual flow. I could think of only one explanation for this TCM diagnosis of Heat as a cause of heavy menstrual bleeding. The ancients might have observed pelvic inflammatory disease where there is an infection in the fallopian tubes with fever, pain, and heavy bleeding. Before antibiotics, cold-cleansing herbs might have been used to treat such infections. In the age of antibiotics, treating with cold-cleansing herbs is no longer warranted. Cold herbs can dilate blood vessels, resulting in a lowered blood pressure. If used on patients who were bleeding heavily, such treatment could potentially put them into shock.

While I have often treated menstrual irregularities in my integrated practice, I have never found a need to use the mobilizing-Blood or cooling-Blood treatment principles recommended in TCM textbooks. I feel that they are inappropriate and potentially dangerous. If the cause was hormonal imbalance and the bleeding was profuse, I prescribed hormones to control the bleeding quickly. I then used tonifying Kidney and tonifying Blood herbs to restore natural hormonal balance and replenish the blood. If blood tests showed anemia, I would also prescribe iron pills. If I were to choose herbs to control bleeding, I would choose hemostatic herbs such as Folium Artemisiae Argyi 艾葉 and tonifying Blood herbs like Gelatinum Asini 阿膠, Angelica Sinensis 當歸, and Polygoni Multiflori 首烏.

Another inappropriate use of mobilizing Qi and Blood herbs is ingesting them for sprains, strains, and traumatic bruising. I have seen patients who received this treatment from TCM practitioners actually have side effects such as bloody urine often seen with too high a dose of anticoagulants like coumadin. While using such herbs in liniment form for such conditions is appropriate, ingesting them can be dangerous.

TCM explains diabetes as Yin deficiency (dehydration) caused by Stomach Heat. Ancient practitioners must have seen the diuretic effect of high blood glucose levels where copious volumes of water and electrolytes were lost in the urine leading to dehydration. Insulin, of course, had not been discovered at the time. If this teaching were followed, only treating Yin deficiency for diabetes would result in delaying insulin treatment. Again, I would warn against tenaciously adhering to inappropriate treatment based on the wrong premise.

The Western treatment of congestive heart failure is undergoing change. Diuresis to minimize the fluid volume the heart needs to pump has remained the same, but Western medicine has been shifting its approach away from treating with positive inotropes (drugs that strengthen heart muscle contraction) to beta-blockers. Beta-blockers make the heart beat less vigorously and more slowly in order to minimize its workload. The TCM approach has not made this shift. Radix Ginseng 人參 might be prescribed according to the older idea of strengthening heart muscle contraction. This approach might overwork the heart, as opposed to the beta-blocker approach, which spares the heart.

Modern drugs have supplanted some old remedies with potential toxicities. These include Cinnabar 朱砂 for febrile convulsions, Gypsum 石膏 for fever, and Talc 滑 for kidney stones. Here, the risks outweigh the benefits.

Often I am asked whether there might be herb-drug interactions when patients taking drugs choose to take TCM remedies also. We must keep in mind that natural products do have medicinal properties. In fact, many of our present day drugs are derived from plants. Aspirin is derived from willow, digitalis from foxglove, birth control pills from yam, the anticancer drug Vincristine from periwinkle, and Taxol from the Pacific yew tree. When combining drugs and herbs, to avoid double dosing, we must be cognizant of the medicinal properties of the herbs. Patients taking the following drugs need to be especially cautious: diuretics, antihypertensives, blood thinners, and antiarrhythmics. Some commonly used herbs have similar actions. This became evident when a Chinese patient came to me for treatment of leg edema and fatigue. She told me that she was on no medications. On her first visit, I found hypertension and some leg edema. As part of my routine studies, I ordered blood electrolytes and found that she had a low serum potassium level. A common cause of low potassium is diuretic therapy, but I had not yet prescribed any diuretics. A rare condition called hyperaldosteronism can also cause low serum potassium. A test I ordered for this condition showed she did not have it. It then occurred to me to ask if she had seen an herbalist for her edema. She said she had. I concluded that the herbalist most likely treated her with diuretic herbs. Just as low potassium can be a side effect of diuretic drugs, it can also be a side effect of diuretic herbs.

A Chinese American psychiatric social worker told me that in the psychiatric ward of his hospital, doctors have become very leery of Chinese herbs. They saw how Chinese patients diagnosed with bipolar mood disorder who had been stabilized with psychiatric drugs rapidly become manic when well-meaning relatives brought them tonifying (Yang) soups. This also occurred when young Chinese women patients with bipolar disorder were brought various concoctions containing Angelica Sinensis 當歸 by their mothers. These herbs tend to be warm and Yang. When combined with antidepressants, also Yang in nature, they can swing a mood disorder excessively toward mania.

Herb-drug interactions are less likely when treating respiratory problems and arthritic conditions because the herbs and drugs used for treating these conditions do not act in the same ways. For bronchodilation, Western drugs tend to stimulate the sympathetic system, which tends to dilate bronchial tubes in preparation for fight or flight. The side effects are from sympathetic stimulation, such as fast heartbeat and tremors. Chinese herbs to help lower lung Qi lack these side effects, so they do not work on the sympathetic system. For arthritis, Western drugs act by blocking the production of prostaglandin, a mediator of inflammation. Chinese herbs for arthritis tend to improve circulation to help the body remove cytokines, the byproducts of inflammation.

How to Use Eastern Medicine

Up to this point, my discussion of Eastern treatments has fallen within the Western paradigm. The focus is on disease. It is important when using Eastern treatments, however, to remember that a major tenet of TCM is to focus not just on the disease but also on the patient and his or her environment. If we simply incorporate Eastern remedies into our Western system, we limit their usefulness.

The Western misapplication of TCM reminds me of a story an old Canadian missionary in Taiwan once told me. For years, the village she lived in had no indoor plumbing, only outhouses with a hole in the ground. Finally, in the early 1970s, she acquired indoor plumbing with an actual toilet with a seat. She was very excited and showed it to a local villager, inviting the villager to try it. "Well, how did you like it?" the missionary asked. To her surprise, the villager answered, "It's a bother, and I don't like it very well." The explanation became obvious when the missionary looked and saw two footprints on the toilet seat.

Some investigators search for and extract the active ingredients in some Chinese herbs to treat disease. Years ago, Dr. K., my ACTCM teacher who had a Western surgical background, told me that Japanese researchers tried just that. They found that using the extracted active ingredients of herbs did not achieve the same effect as when the same herbs were used in a traditional Chinese prescription. The reason for this shortcoming is that these researchers left the patient out of the picture.

In an Australian controlled study on the efficacy of an herbal formula to treat menopausal symptoms, fifty-five postmenopausal women all received the same formula, and then a survey was taken to compare the effect of the herb formula with a placebo. The study concluded that the herb formula was no better than the placebo (Davis, et al. 2001). The problem is that the controlled study assumed that if the subjects were the same age and sex, and had similar health conditions, they were alike. A true TCM study would at least recognize that certain women had certain imbalances, and would sort them into groups to account for the imbalances.

In contrast, an Eastern model was used in another Australian study on the efficacy of Chinese herbal medicine on irritable bowel syndrome. In this study, a TCM practitioner diagnosed each patient and prescribed herbal treatment according to TCM principles. Sorted out this way, the TCM treatments were found to be effective (Bensoussan, et al. 1998).

My friend Pamela, a nurse, told me she was eating large quantities of carrots for beta-carotene, a known antioxidant. I warned her that the Chinese consider carrots to belong to the cool category of foods and that large quantities might be harmful. I later read a study that showed the use of beta-carotene in lung cancer patients actually hastened their deaths (The Alpha-Tocopheral Beta Carotene Cancer Prevention Study Group 1994). This was an enigma to Western researchers, since other studies show beta-carotene to be a preventive against cancer (Cooper, et al. 1999). The Eastern practitioner would explain that beta-carotene treatment could not be applied in a vacuum, without consideration of the patient's overall balance. A patient's immune system might be too deficient. Treatment with a cold-type substance like beta-carotene would further lower the patient's immune response against the cancer. This may well be why many of our double-blind and age-sex matched controlled studies yield conflicting results. These studies assume that a group of matched subjects is homogenous.

We can be misled even in our evidence-based studies if we ignore the genetic and environmental factors influencing health (see chapter 8). In the 1970s, I worked in an English-speaking mission clinic in Taipei, Taiwan. Those were the days before plastic syringes and vacuum test tubes. Blood was drawn using glass syringes and then transferred to test tubes. The ancillary help, such as X-ray technicians and lab technicians, lacked the customary credentials required in the West. They were trained on the job. One day, I happened to be in the lab and saw that the technician had left a glass syringe filled with blood on the countertop. I told her to quickly empty the syringe into a test tube because the blood left in the glass syringe would quickly clot, making it impossible to transfer. She said, "Oh, don't worry, Dr. Tsang, this is Chinese blood. It will not clot. If it were Caucasian blood, I would transfer it into test tubes immediately because, as you said, it will clot. However, Chinese blood will not. See." She proceeded to show me that, indeed, the Chinese blood that had been sitting in the glass syringe for fifteen minutes was still in liquid form as she transferred it into the test tube. Indeed, we are not all the same. There are genetic, constitutional, and environmental differences.

With cancer therapy, mainstream medicine has begun to recognize that individuals with the same disease do not all respond to the same drugs in the same way. They came to this realization when using expensive and potentially dangerous chemotherapeutic agents. They discovered that response to drugs was genetically determined. Individual responders could be sorted out by studying their genetic makeup. This approach is called pharmacogenomics (National Center for Biotechnology Information 2004). Allopathic medicine has finally realized that each patient is unique, something TCM has understood for a long time.

Pauline was a nurse in her thirties who saw me for headaches, sleep disturbance, and some bodily aches and pains. After a series of herbal and acupuncture therapies, she recovered, and I did not see her for six months. One day she returned with a recurrence of all her symptoms. When I asked her what happened, she told me she had read about the benefits of Ginkgo Bilobae, and she began taking large quantities of the herb. I asked Dr. Lai whether Ginkgo was as beneficial as Westerners considered it to be. He said that Chinese practitioners do not consider it a particularly valuable herb. It is meant to be used in small quantities, either in cooking or as a small part of an herbal prescription. It was never meant to be consumed the way Americans are consuming it. In fact, a textbook on Chinese herbs states that Ginkgo in high doses is toxic. Toxic manifestations include headache, fever, tremors, irritability, and dyspnea (shortness of breath) (Bensky 1987, 560).

Ginkgo has been touted to have antiplatelet and procirculatory therapeutic effects, but Dr. Lai said that many herbs in the TCM pharmacopoeia are far superior to Ginkgo for dispersing and vitalizing blood. He pointed out that herbs sold on the open market in Asia are like U.S. commodities: when the herb is valuable and scarce, it commands a high price. Ginkgo Bilobae has never commanded a high price in Asia. Pauline's case demonstrated to me the danger for Westerners who use components of Eastern remedies with a Western approach without considering how these remedies fit into the Eastern paradigm. The result may be further imbalance.

Weight reduction is an area in which herbs are the most misused. Aristolochia Fangchi 馬兜鈴, sometimes used in diet pills, has been reported to cause nephropathy and kidney cancer (Nortier, et al. 2000). This herb was meant to be used only in small doses and for a brief course for coughs. It was never meant to be used on a long-term basis or for weight reduction.

The Importance of the TCM Paradigm

Our curiosity about TCM and our enthusiasm for its remedies must be tempered with care and caution. There is a proper and an improper way to use TCM remedies. The correct way requires using treatments within the TCM paradigm.

The Ben 本 (Root)

"The patient was well until two weeks ago when he developed …"
This is a very common opening phrase found in medical histories.
They usually record the present problem as having begun when
acute symptoms began. Was the patient really well until only two
weeks ago? Careful history-taking will point a TCM practitioner
to an event that gradually threw the patient's homeostasis off balance far earlier, but the transition can be so subtle that the patient
failed to notice the change. Often the practitioner needs to ferret
it out of the patient. In my integrated practice, whenever I probed
regarding the onset of an illness, patients often related the onset of
their symptoms to a particular event. "It started when my second
child was born … It started after my car accident … It started in my
second year of college." The common thread in their stories is that
the patient was enjoying good health until some stressor tipped
the balance, causing the body's homeostatic mechanism to lose its
equilibrium. The Western medical paradigm, lacking the concept
of Ben 本, focuses only on the Biao 表 or the external manifestation
of an imbalance. TCM teaches that if we merely treat the present-
ing problem (the Biao 表), there is often incomplete resolution of
the problem. We need to find and treat the underlying imbalance
(the root 本) that led to the problem in order to restore the patient
to true wellness. This approach distinguishes TCM from allopathic
medicine. It is no wonder that when Westerners use a TCM remedy that treats the Biao 表, they find it ineffective. The prevalent
mainstream Western belief that all complementary treatments
must undergo evidence based investigation to be deemed effective
has missed this important aspect of the Eastern paradigm. The
evidence focuses on treating disease, not the patient.

When Jean came to see me for iritis, an autoimmune condition in which the body inappropriately attacks the eye, she was
forty-nine. Her doctor had ordered an HLA-B27 antigen test, which
was positive. This meant she was genetically prone to certain
types of autoimmune conditions like iritis. Her ophthalmologist

prescribed steroid eye drops, which helped the eye inflammation, but as soon as she stopped the drops, the iritis recurred. She had been treated by two other TCM practitioners who prescribed cooling herbs for the eye inflammation. The concoctions made her feel weak and lightheaded without improving her eye inflammation. Noting her age, I asked her about signs of menopause, such as hot flashes, palpitations, sleep disturbance, and menstrual irregularities. Of those symptoms, she had palpitations and irregular periods. For six months before the onset of her iritis, her periods were extremely heavy. During that time, she had palpitations and her doctor ordered a treadmill test, which was normal.

I did a TCM analysis of Jean's case. Her positive HLA-B27 test indicates that she has a genetic predisposition for iritis. She had not developed iritis until age forty-eight, at the onset of menopause when her Kidney Qi was declining. Her heavy periods meant she was Blood deficient. Her palpitations meant she had Deficient Liver Fire (see chapter 2) resulting from menstrual blood loss. My prescriptions for her included herbs not only to calm the eye inflammation (the Biao 表) but also herbs to tonify Blood and Kidney Qi (the Ben 本), and herbs to calm Deficient Liver Fire. With that type of herb prescription, her iritis resolved, she was able to stop the steroid drops, and her palpitations stopped. Despite her genetic predisposition, Jean's body had been able to keep iritis at bay for forty-eight years. The blood loss and decline of hormonal balance with menopause tipped the balance for her. The steroid eye drops and cooling herbs treated only the Biao 表, the iritis. Jean improved only when her Blood deficiency and Kidney Qi deficiency, the Ben 本, were addressed.

The Economics of Energy

The economics of energy is another concept that distinguishes the Eastern from the Western medical paradigm. In 1998, I attended a lecture given by Dr. Rajesh Munglani, a pain management consultant. He spoke about an animal research study that had astonishing results and implications. Normally with an injury, chemicals at the spinal cord level send pain-stimulating messages up to the brain. The brain responds by sending pain-suppressing messages down the spinal cord to neutralize the pain-stimulating chemicals. Munglani, et al. (1996) found that even after the injury had healed, when the animal appeared normal and exhibited no increased sensitivity to painful stimulation, there were still pain-suppressing chemicals found in its spinal cord, indicating that the body remained in an adaptive mode.

Extrapolating this finding to humans, you could say that after an injury, when the wound appears healed and the patient appears to have recovered, the patient's brain may still be in an adaptive mode, giving only the illusion of complete recovery. This tells me that homeostasis requires hard work and energy. We are normal because our bodies are constantly at work to maintain the status quo. If an extra workload is placed on it, the body might not have enough energy to compensate for the increased burden.

Often patients who have had multiple surgeries still have the pain the surgery was supposed to have cured. Their scars are well healed, the various scans and X-rays show no evidence of the former problem, but the symptoms fail to resolve. It could be that their bodies' powers of adaptation have just become exhausted. One such patient reported that after surgery, she had not improved. She then tried various other kinds of treatments such as physical therapy and chiropractics. The only thing that seemed to help her was an herbal concoction prescribed by a TCM practitioner to tonify her various deficiencies.

The results of this animal research study could also explain why so many chronic conditions flare when patients become tired or lack adequate sleep. A patient of mine had been in a car accident. Right after, she developed acute double vision because the impact injured the nerve supplying the muscle to one eye. With time, she noticed the double vision resolved, but it sometimes returned when she was tired. Recognizing that there is an economics to our internal energy allocation, TCM approaches the problem by using herbs to add energy when it runs low.

Gearing Treatment to Stages of Disease

Disease evolves in stages. The skeptics who scoff at complementary medicine because it treats patients who are "not very sick" inadvertently diagnosed the problem with allopathic medicine: allopathic treatments are mainly geared for the very sick, but we have far fewer treatments for patients who suffer from early stages of a disease. That truth also explains why Western health care tends to be costly. TCM methods are more effective in early, mild, or chronic stages because they try to detect and treat imbalances in the host to enable self-healing. When conditions become acute or severe, Western methods, which tend to take over or replace bodily functions, are needed.

With conditions such as asthma, Western drugs can be life saving for the acute severe stage. After the patient becomes stabilized, Chinese herbs can be introduced to help reduce the dosage of asthma drugs with their inherent side effects, and, sometimes, drugs can even be discontinued. I would, however, warn against abrupt discontinuation of drugs when just beginning TCM treatment. Response to TCM treatments tends to be gradual. The patient must show improvement before drugs are tapered, and they should be discontinued only if improvement is maintained. It is unfortunate that many Chinese patients regard Chinese herbs and Western drugs to be always incompatible. This misconception can be traced back to the past when Eastern and Western practitioners were more polarized. In order to protect their respective turf, they instilled the fear in patients of dire consequences from mixing the two kinds of remedies. Sadly, I have seen patients inappropriately discontinue needed maintenance drugs such as antihypertensives when they began herbal therapy for such conditions as colds and the flu.

For peripheral vascular disease, the Western treatment is surgical bypass when disease is in an advanced stage. For cases not yet requiring bypass, Western medicine resorts to watchful waiting. Allopathic remedies such as pentoxifylline are not effective, whereas herbs are often effective in improving circulation to the limbs and can forestall the need for surgery.

For degenerative arthritis of large joints, before the advanced stages when surgical replacement is required, again, the Western approach is watchful waiting. Drugs such as nonsteroidal anti-inflammatories for pain relief carry risk. Acupuncture and herbal remedies can relieve symptoms and also forestall the need for surgery.

For patients with coronary heart disease, Western preventive measures such as diet, low-dose aspirin, and cholesterol-lowering drugs are effective mainstays. An adjunct to this regimen could be herbs that also discourage plaque formation. If a coronary artery is more than 90 percent blocked, though, life-saving surgical procedures like angioplasty or coronary artery bypass are needed. After surgery and during convalescence, herbs can be resumed to help hasten recovery and again be an adjunct in preventing further plaque formation.

For diabetes, no one can deny the benefits of Western drugs. Insulin has saved many lives. Newer drugs are now available to help patients who are not insulin dependent, but those drugs still have limitations (see chapter 9). Certain Spleen herbs can be used as adjuncts to drugs for type 2 diabetes.

Many Western drugs actually are directed at interfering with normal functions. Our pharmacopeias are replete with drugs that either block or inhibit: SSRI-type antidepressants are selective serotonin reuptake inhibitors; drugs for acid reflux, also known as PPIs, are proton pump inhibitors. Cheryl Schwartz, a doctor of veterinary medicine who pioneered using TCM for treating animals, writes in the introduction to her book, *Four Paws, Five Directions*, that she found most of her treatments consisted of prescribing antibiotics and anti-inflammatories. In fact, all of her treatments seemed "anti-something" (1996). NSAIDs, for instance, block the production of prostaglandins, which cause inflammation. Antibiotics interfere with a microorganism's ability to multiply, but they are taken internally and can affect the host as well. Drugs can be effective in the short term, to quickly resolve an acute condition. But in the long term, when we interfere with normal function, other problems will emerge. For chronic conditions, a complementary approach such as TCM is preferable.

The difference in philosophic influences between East and West has caused their medical paradigms to develop along divergent paths. The West, with its emphasis on analysis, has furthered the understanding of disease processes and refined ways to diagnose and treat using a targeted approach. The East, with its emphasis on wholeness, has directed attention to ways to enhance the host's ability to fight disease and stay balanced. Ideally, the two approaches can be used to complement one another; this can be done best when there is an understanding of both.

"An invasion of armies can be resisted, but not an idea whose time has come."

— Victor Hugo

Chapter 15
TCM and Our Future

I n America, we are facing a health-care crisis of colossal proportions. Many factors are at play. The political and economic interests
that fuel this problem notwithstanding, my discussion will address
it as if our interests were all aligned—to benefit the patient. In part,
we are the victims of our progress. Increased life expectancy has
added $20,000 to the cost of health care for each person per year. All
would agree that we should maximize prevention, early detection,
and intervention, and minimize risk and cost. How can Eastern
medicine help us achieve these goals?

Training

Progress often comes at a price. The information age has given
rise to identity theft; pesticides have led to pollution; the digital
age has given rise to a new disease called repetitive strain injury.
With tremendous advances in medical technology, we are also
paying a price not only in the matter of high health-care costs
but also in the gradual erosion of clinical skills among recently
trained physicians. The trend is to rely heavily on technology.
The mainstays of taking a history and doing a thorough physical

examination have fallen by the wayside. In the 1990s, I performed a physical examination on a twenty-three-year-old woman. When I palpated for her heart on the left side of the chest, I could not feel the usual heartbeat. Further tests showed that she had situs inversus, a condition from birth in which the heart is on the right side of the chest rather than on the left. She marveled that despite having seen a number of pediatricians and gynecologists in her twenty-three years, no other physician had found her abnormality. Physical diagnosis is currently not given the emphasis it deserves in our training programs.

Recently, I have observed how modern technology has sometimes impeded rather than enhanced health care. One friend's appendicitis ruptured because of a four-hour wait for a CT scan. Another friend's intestinal obstruction was missed by an ER physician who discharged her because her abdominal ultrasound was normal. I made the diagnosis by listening to her history over the phone, confirmed it with a focused abdominal exam, and advised her to try another ER. At the second ER, diagnosis and treatment were delayed for three hours pending the result of a CT scan. I have witnessed physicians in mainstream hospitals miss diagnoses of appendicitis, hepatic carcinoma, and congestive heart failure. CT scans and MRIs are invaluable tools, but they should not replace clinical evaluation of the patient.

One glaring deficiency in Western medical training is in the physical diagnosis of musculoskeletal soft tissue maladies. Too often, the automatic response to such problems is to order MRIs without a thorough hands-on examination. Patients who consulted me for acupuncture liked to give me details of all the tests other doctors had ordered. Rarely were the test results helpful. What was most helpful was to listen to their stories: how the problem began, how it progressed, what made it improve, what made it worse, and how it limited function. Next in importance was a thorough examination, including not only palpating for muscle tension, tenderness, and range of motion, but also skin changes in the affected area.

Mark came to see me for acupuncture. While crossing the street, he had been hit by a car and thrown twenty feet. He was in his early forties and had been otherwise in excellent health. After the injury, he suffered from debilitating back pain. Because his MRIs were normal, the attorneys defending the driver who hit him deemed his injuries insignificant. His case went to court. The orthopedist who testified as an expert witness offered no objective findings to strengthen Mark's case. The opposing attorney portrayed Mark as a malingerer. When I took the stand, I pointed out the one sign indicating that Mark's pain was real. I had learned from a course on intramuscular stimulation that one sign of neuropathy was excessive localized sweating. Whenever I examined Mark's back prior to acupuncture treatments, I observed profuse sweating over the specific location of his lumbar back pain. With that bit of evidence, the tables turned, and Mark won the case.

If we are to alter the costly path of modern medicine, we need to begin by redirecting how we train physicians. Before we had CT and MRI capabilities, physicians were trained to focus on the patient and use every noninvasive means to arrive at a diagnosis. TCM physicians went further because they lacked even labs and X-rays. TCM diagnosis is high in sensitivity but low in specificity. Using observation with pulse and tongue examination, Chinese practitioners can detect early imbalances in a region of the body at a very early stage of disease, but they are unable to pinpoint the exact location or specific nature of the problem. Western technology can pinpoint problems very specifically. Ideally, we should combine the sensitivity of the East with the specificity of the West. If we stretch our imaginations, perhaps we can even adapt our technology to detect early changes in the pulse that TCM practitioners have been trained to do after years of training and experience.

In California, physicians are now required to receive twelve hours of terminal care and pain-management training to maintain licensure. To meet these requirements, I attended two courses. In the first, palliative-care specialists taught how to use narcotic analgesics to manage pain in terminally ill patients. In the second course, I was appalled to find that pain-management experts in mainstream medicine recommended using narcotic analgesics for chronic musculoskeletal pain. Teaching physicians to use narcotics to manage pain in the terminally ill is appropriate, but teaching primary care doctors to use narcotics for chronic musculoskeletal pain is inappropriate and does society a great disservice. When we consider risk/benefit ratios, the risks of both NSAIDs and narcotics far outweigh their benefits when compared to acupuncture, yet acupuncture is not even mentioned in current pain-management curricula. One lecturer lamented that the public showed more interest in complementary therapies for neuropathic pain than the conventional allopathic drug approach he was teaching. The public should be commended for using common sense.

Research

In the area of research, the media has bedazzled Westerners regarding the potentials of Eastern medicine. This has misled us into doing research in inconsequential areas. Qi gong and acupuncture anesthesia for surgery sound beguiling, but do we need them? Only skilled masters can perform Qi gong properly. If used incorrectly, it can have harmful effects. How many can this ancient art benefit? As for acupuncture anesthesia, even in China, it is used in only 20 percent of cases, and patients are carefully selected. Only those with high pain thresholds are candidates. That criterion would eliminate most pampered Westerners. Often when I read in the newspapers about "new" discoveries in medicine, I am disappointed. Usually, the medical community has known about most of these so-called new developments for about a decade. We live in a global community. When NIH pronounced in 1995 that acupuncture might be effective for certain kinds of pain and for nausea, I could imagine our neighbors across the ocean asking, "Are they trying to reinvent the wheel?" Such information has been common knowledge not for years or decades but for millennia. The effectiveness of acupuncture for painful musculoskeletal conditions is common knowledge to acupuncturists and patients alike. In the pain management course I recently attended, the lecturer stated that because of their long established use, there was no need for controlled double blind studies to determine if narcotic drugs were effective for pain. That argument is even more applicable to acupuncture. As early as the nineteenth century in America, William Osler, considered the father of modern medicine, recommended acupuncture for treatment of back pain.

Research involves having a hypothesis, asking a question about whether the hypothesis is correct, and then proceeding to investigate for the answer. We in the west are squandering our resources by asking outdated questions. In the words of the famous American bank robber Willie Sutton, let us go "where the money is."

Acupuncture

In 1971, when the *New York Times* reporter James Reston underwent emergency appendectomy while visiting Beijing and then was treated for postoperative pain with acupuncture, it made front-page news. We are ready for the next headline news: "Acupuncture cures appendicitis." Existing Chinese studies show that the acupuncture point, Stomach 36, located in the vicinity of the lateral sural cutaneous nerve, the cutaneous branch of the saphenous nerve, and the deep peroneal nerve, can influence gastrointestinal motility and also improve immune function (O'Connor 1981, 529). We should be asking the question, "How is that possible?" Are there autonomic nerves accompanying the nerves at this acupuncture point that we have yet to map? Is the mechanism antidromic nerve conduction? How can needling a point on the leg influence the immune system? Does it cause release of hormones to stimulate the bone marrow or thymus gland or lymph nodes?

Chinese studies have shown that stimulating Stomach 36 and another point below it, called MLE 13 (Lanweixue), can regulate peristalsis in the appendix leading to passage of an impacted fecolith

(O'Connor 1981). At present, if a patient sees a physician for right lower abdominal pain, appendicitis is the diagnosis to be considered. The treatment of choice is surgery. We examine the patient and order laboratory tests. If the pain is typical but our examination and tests do not show acute inflammation, we have the patient rest, restrict oral intake to fluids, and return for reexamination. Because the treatment is invasive and carries risk, we wait for signs that the appendix is actually inflamed before proceeding with surgery. During this period of watchful waiting, the Western approach lacks any measures to reverse the process. This is the gap that acupuncture can fill. Although acupuncture will not eliminate the need for surgery in all cases, we should investigate the possibility of its benefiting cases that are in the early stages.

Other Chinese studies show that stimulating GB 34 improves gallbladder function and facilitates flow through the biliary tract. Just as for early appendicitis, we can investigate how this information can benefit treatment of gallstones. Chinese studies also show that stimulating St 36, GB 34, and Li 3 can relieve morphine-induced spasms in the sphincter of Oddi (O'Connor 1981, 530). The sphincter of Oddi is the muscular ring controlling the ampulla of Vater, the common channel for bile and pancreatic juices to flow through on the way to the small intestines. Sometimes gallstones can obstruct the flow. The backed-up bile and digestive juices seep into the pancreas, setting up an intense inflammatory reaction called pancreatitis. Western treatment consists of pain medication, putting the digestive tract to rest by suctioning out stomach juices, intravenous fluids, and watchful waiting. When gallstones are suspected of obstructing the common bile duct or ampulla of Vater, gastroenterologists often use a procedure called ERCP to cut the smooth muscles of the sphincter of Oddi to widen the opening for the gallstones to pass. If acupuncture can relax the sphincter of Oddi, it may sometimes eliminate the need for cutting it.

There is evidence that stimulation of UB 67 located on the sural nerve in the foot can induce rotation of a breech presentation of the fetus in obstetrics. We should be asking, "How does this work? Can we save some costly C-sections using this method for breech presentations?"

The cost of infertility testing and treatment has reached stratospheric levels. As mentioned earlier, common experience tells us that TCM, by using both acupuncture and herbs, has a definite role in treating the problem of infertility. We could consider TCM as a first option for infertile couples before embarking on the expensive high tech route. There is room for the West to learn how China became the most populous country on the planet.

Western studies show that stimulation of Spleen 6 on the posterior tibial nerve can affect genitourinary function. These studies came about because urologists had tried to find ways to control bladder dysfunction by implanting various electrodes into the spinal cord and nerves that directly control detrusor muscle function (the muscle responsible for voiding). The problem was that patients could not tolerate the discomfort of these procedures. The urologists then thought of adopting the idea from acupuncture of stimulating the posterior tibial nerve that was easily accessible in the lower leg to achieve their end and found that it was as effective as their other more invasive techniques. Other Western researchers are similarly studying ways to control nervous dysfunction and chronic pain by implanting electrodes in the spinal cord. These procedures carry risk and are expensive. They could likewise borrow ideas from acupuncture to achieve these ends.

Herbal Therapy

Cardiovascular disease ranks high in research priorities of western countries. From firsthand clinical experience, I know that combinations of herbs in the quelling-Wind and mobilizing-Qi-and-Blood categories can influence peripheral vascular disease. Yet when I tried to apply for a grant with NIH to study the effect of herbs for peripheral vascular disease, I was told that the funding for complementary care research had been used up to study the effect of massage therapy on HIV-AIDS.

As I mentioned in chapter 3, we are made of a network of tubes or ducts. Mobilizing-Qi herbs function by relaxing the smooth muscles that make up the walls of ducts. In addition to using them to treat vascular disease, we can use them to treat conditions in which ducts are obstructed, such as in the case of kidney stones, gallstones, and salivary duct stones.

Obesity and type 2 diabetes mellitus are major concerns in developed and developing countries. We should ask some questions about the role of Spleen herbs in addressing these issues. Do they work by decreasing insulin resistance? Do they enhance incretin secretion? Are they useful for controlling obesity? Certain acupuncture points are also known to help lower blood glucose levels. We certainly have not exhausted the possibilities offered by TCM in these areas.

There is widespread misunderstanding in both Eastern and Western thinking regarding the role of TCM in cancer therapy. Many Chinese believe that the patient needs to avoid nourishing food and tonifying herbs to prevent the cancer cells from proliferating. The reality is that starving the cancer cells simultaneously starves the host and impairs his or her ability to fight the cancer. Chinese cancer patients often have the misconception that if Western chemotherapy offers only palliation and no hope of cure, they are better off turning to herbal therapy alone for cure. This either/or thinking is flawed. When even early stage cancer has been diagnosed, the cancer has already been growing for a long time—a matter of years. The presence of cancer cells represents a failure of the host's own body to contain tumor growth. The TCM approach works best in early stage disease. To rely on herbs alone for a cure of a disease that can no longer be considered early is unrealistic. On the other side, many Western practitioners prohibit patients from taking herbal therapy, mainly because the effects are unknown to them. Yet there is little effort among Westerners to investigate the role of herbs.

Chinese herbal therapy can play two roles in cancer therapy. One is to ameliorate the devastating side effects of Western therapy. Many Yin tonifying herbs can restore moisture to dry mucous membranes. Tonifying Kidney and Spleen herbs can help with the debilitating fatigue of Western cancer therapy. After a course of chemotherapy or radiation, there is a watch-and-wait period when the patient doesn't receive treatment but is monitored for recurrence. It is during this period that Chinese herbal therapy plays a second role. Some Chinese herbs have antitumor properties. Two common ones are Oldenlandie Diffusae 白花蛇舌草 and Ganoderma Lucidum and Ganoderma Since 靈芝. More studies are needed. Such herbs in a prescription balanced with immune-boosting herbs could be considered for maintenance anticancer therapy. We are well aware of the toll Western cancer therapy takes on patients' well-being. There is a need to study the potential benefits of adding Eastern treatments.

Currently Western medicine has shown intense interest in the immune system. In this area, Eastern methods trump Western ones. Certain acupuncture points and herbs that tonify Spleen and Kidney actually enhance the immune response. Western drugs usually only suppress the response. Let us consider autoimmune diseases, conditions in which the body inappropriately mounts an immune response to its own tissues. Our experience with the HIV-AIDS epidemic should have taught us a lesson about autoimmunity. Early in the epidemic, before there were antiretroviral drugs, we saw the natural progression of this deadly disease. It was common for HIV-AIDS patients, people with extremely weak immune systems, to develop autoimmune diseases. Logic would tell us that autoimmune diseases arise from a weakened, malfunctioning immune system. Knowing this, we should question our allopathic approach of using drugs such as steroids and antimetabolites that further suppress the immune response in autoimmune diseases. The immune system is extremely complex, consisting not only of cells that attack foreign invaders but also of other cells that direct what to attack. A portion of this system, called self-nonself recognition, specifically prevents attacks on one's own tissues (Jiang and Chess 2006). When functioning normally, this component prevents autoimmune diseases. The Western approach of suppressing the entire immune system discounts the importance of the Yin-Yang balance in a functioning immune system. The Eastern approach strengthens the entire immune system and allows spontaneous rebalance of its various components.

Researchers have found that conditions in which there is prolonged inflammation are associated with cancer. Lung cancer can develop from benign-appearing scars that are the aftermath of pulmonary tuberculosis. In the case of latent tuberculosis, the immune system is constantly at work to contain the tuberculosis bacilli that years before gained entry into the body. In these cases, when immunity becomes compromised, such as with steroid treatment, tuberculosis can become reactivated. Colon cancer is more prevalent in patients who have the autoimmune disease ulcerative colitis, an inflammatory condition. Recent studies have focused on using anti-inflammatories to prevent colon cancer, but because of the serious deleterious effects of anti-inflammatories on the cardiovascular system, this approach has been abandoned (Bresalier, et al. 2005). If we think of the TCM concept of economics of energy, we should ask these two questions: Could it be that in these cases so much immune energy is directed at inflammation that the immune system becomes depleted and its function of surveillance against tumor cells become compromised? Could immune boosting with acupuncture and tonifying Spleen or Kidney herbs, in addition to antioxidants and diet control, have a role in prevention?

Up to now, Eastern and Western medicine have been entrenched in "us and them" camps. Even when Western practitioners pay lip service to complementary care as a viable option for their patients, they still view "them" as having strange, unintelligible ideas based on mysticism; as having treatments that, while sometimes effective, can't be scientifically proven. Therefore comparing "them" on an equal footing with "us" in the allopathic camp is just untenable. Western practitioners of Chinese descent are particularly suspicious of TCM. Perhaps it is because they have seen the disastrous results when Chinese patients have triaged themselves, seeking TCM treatment inappropriately and getting Western help too late. Perhaps they have seen appendixes rupture or cancers progress to become inoperable. Eastern practitioners view Western ways as harmful. They view surgery as something to avoid at all costs and drugs as having toxic side effects and being incompatible with herbal therapy. It is my hope that this book will dispel some of these long-held notions and open dialogue between East and West in order to achieve optimal healing.

Glossary

ACTCM American College of Traditional Chinese Medicine

Addison's disease a disease characterized by darkened skin, severe prostration, anemia, low blood pressure, diarrhea, and digestive disturbance caused by failure of the adrenal gland

adrenergic activated or transmitted by adrenaline

allergen a substance inducing an allergic response

anatomic pertaining to bodily structure

ankylosing spondylitis a disease characterized by fusion of the entire spine

antiplatelet causing platelets to not adhere to one another and thereby lessening the tendency for blood to clot

atrial fibrillation an abnormal heart rhythm that causes the heart to beat inefficiently and that sometimes results in abnormal clotting in the heart chamber. A clot can then potentially break off, pass to the brain, and result in a stroke.

autoimmune disease a disease characterized by the body's immune system attacking the body's own tissue

baseline function any bodily function at rest before the onset of an illness

Bei a TCM term describing an arthritic condition in which it is felt there is blockage of Qi

Ben the original root cause of a disease believed in TCM to be an imbalance in one of the eight dualities, an organ dysfunction, or a depletion of a bodily substance

beta-blocker a class of drugs that block the receptors (beta receptors) to beta-adrenergic stimulation. The result is lowered bodily response to adrenergic stimulation.

Biao the external manifestation of a root problem. In TCM, the symptom or sign that the patient presents is only the tip of the iceberg, the Biao. Treating it is not adequate to cure the patient. In addition to the Biao, the TCM practitioner must find the Ben.

Blood deficiency a TCM term equivalent to blood loss. There is not only loss of red blood cells (anemia) but also a depletion of the fluid part of the blood. In TCM, both need to be replenished.

Blood Stasis a TCM term that includes not only problems with abnormally clotted blood but also ecchymosis or bruising

Burners (Upper, Middle, and Lower) three regions of the body. The upper burner is the region above the diaphragm, the middle is the abdominal viscera, and the lower is the genitourinary tract and lower extremities.

Calming liver (or calming liver fire) to decrease sympathetic and adrenergic activity

carpal tunnel syndrome a syndrome characterized by tingling pain and/or numbness of the palmar aspect of the hand and sometimes pain in the palmar aspect of the wrist caused by compression by swollen soft tissue of the median nerve as it passes through a tunnel-like opening at the wrist. More advanced cases can involve weakness of the muscles moving the thumb.

cervical disc disease a disease of the discs in the neck. Discs all along the spine are resilient shock absorbers sandwiched between the vertebrae. They are made up of an outer fibrous layer and an inner jelly-like substance. When the cervical discs degenerate, there are tears in the fibrous layer, and the inner jelly can seep out and also become dry. The discs then lose their former height. This results in a narrowing of the opening for nerves to exit the spine. Impingement of the nerves in the neck where they exit from the spine to supply the upper extremities results in symptoms of neck pain and numbness or tingling in the arm or hand.

cirrhosis a condition of inflammation, destruction, and regeneration of liver cells leading to abnormal scarring

cluster headaches a type of vascular headache characterized by severe unilateral headaches that occur in a series or clusters within a short period

cortisol major glucocorticoid hormone produced by the adrenal cortex. It is involved in carbohydrate, protein, lipid, and water metabolism.

Coumadin a drug that interferes with the clotting mechanism

cytokines hormones regulating the immune response produced by cells of various tissues

diaphoresis sweating

Dispersing blood blood thinning

diuretic promoting eliminations of fluid by the kidney

double-blind studies a research method in which test subjects are divided into two groups; one receives the treatment to be tested and the other does not, but the two groups are "blinded" so that neither the subjects nor the researchers know who is receiving the treatment

Downbearing function of stomach peristalsis or the function of moving ingested food downward toward the intestines

ecchymosis bruising the accumulation of blood that has escaped from a broken blood vessel and seeped into surrounding tissue. In TCM, ecchymosis is part of blood stasis, which means blood has been prevented from coursing in a normal direction.

edema abnormal accumulation of fluid in the tissues

endometriosis a condition in which the cells that are normally found in the lining of the uterus grow outside their normal location

endorphin a pain-relieving hormone produced in the brain and pituitary gland

epididymitis inflammation of the epididymis, the tube transporting semen in the male genitourinary tract

erythropoietin hormone produced mainly in the kidney and liver that stimulates red blood cell production by the bone marrow

etiology cause of a disease

eustachian tube a tube-like structure connecting the middle ear to the nasopharynx

fecolith dried feces that becomes stone-like and can obstruct the opening of the appendix

feedback mechanism the normal regulatory mechanism for many physiologic functions that shuts off a gland when the level of its secretion has reached a normal level

fibrin a proteinaceous substance that holds a blood clot together

flexion contracture spastic contraction of muscles that flex limbs when counteraction by paralyzed extensor muscles is either too weak or absent as a result of a stroke

FSH follicle-stimulating hormone, a hormone secreted by the pituitary gland to stimulate the ovaries to ovulate

GI gastrointestinal

glaucoma a disease of the eye in which optic nerve cells degenerate, sometimes caused by increased fluid pressure in the eye

glomeruli the kidney's filtering units

glycogen the molecular form glucose takes when stored in the liver

gout a condition caused by abnormal purine metabolism in which uric acid levels are abnormally high and crystallize in tissues causing painful inflammation, commonly in joints

granuloma a mass resulting from the body's reaction, forming fibrous tissue to isolate a foreign substance

homeostasis the body's mechanism of regulating various functions to maintain normality

Hot Qi a condition characterized by dry mouth, halitosis, nosebleeds, acne, and constipation. It represents a relative Yin deficiency.

hyperactive airway disease a condition in which the normal cough reflex is hyperactive, usually as a result of the bronchial airways having been injured in a respiratory infection and the normal mucous and ciliary action inside the bronchi not completely recovering

interferon a cytokine that fights viruses

Internal Heat a stage of an infectious disease in which there is fever. TCM explains that the Cold Evil has penetrated the skin and muscles, and entered the interior organs of the body.

Internal Wind the TCM explanation of the origins of a stroke. TCM explains that wind causes the catastrophic sudden illness; the origin of the wind is not atmospheric but from the interior of the body where there is excessive Liver fire, meaning excessive sympathetic stimulation leading to high blood pressure.

lumbar disc disease like cervical disc disease. The same degenerative process occurs in the lumbar area of the spine, with pinching of the nerves to the legs.

lumbar spinal stenosis a narrowing in the opening in the spinal column where nerves emerge, causing pinching of the nerves supplying the leg and foot

meralgia paresthetica a condition characterized by numbness in the front of the thigh caused by pinching of the lateral cutaneous nerve of the thigh

NSAID nonsteroidal anti-inflammatory drug

norepinephrine the hormone secreted by sympathetic nerves and the adrenal medulla, causing constriction of blood vessels

Painful Wind Chinese name for gout

pancreatitis inflammation of the pancreas

parasympathetic nervous system the part of the autonomic nervous system that stimulates vegetative function such as digestion

peristalsis the normal synchronized movement of the GI tract that propels ingested food and liquid down the GI tract

placebo in a double-blind research study, an imitation of a drug that has no active ingredients. It is given to the half of test subjects not receiving the drug being tested.

plantar fasciitis inflammation of the plantar fascia of the foot, characterized by pain in the sole and heel of the foot

Planted Wind TCM term for stroke

posttraumatic stress disorder a condition in which a person who has undergone severe stress remains in a state of hyperarousal for over a month

prostacyclin a substance made by endothelial cells lining blood vessels that dilates blood vessels and inhibits platelets from adhering to each other. It counterbalances the effects of thromboxane, which has an opposite action.

prostaglandin a substance that is made in various tissues with multiple physiologic effects, one of which is inflammation

Qi a widely used Chinese term literally meaning "air," which, when combined with other words, is used to mean the essential mechanism by which a phenomenon that is not well understood functions

Quelling Wind herbs a group of herbs that have in common the effect of dilating small blood vessels

Raynaud's Phenomenon a condition that involves excessive vaso-constriction of the fingers and toes, especially in the presence of cold temperatures

Relieving Surface herbs See Quelling Wind herbs.

Sjogren's Syndrome an autoimmune disease in which the body attacks fluid-secreting glands, characterized by dry eyes and dry mouth

Solid a TCM term describing the body's physiologic response to infection

sphincter of Oddi a smooth muscle that can contract or dilate to control the flow of bile entering the small intestines

Spleen wetness a condition of excessive fluid retention

steroid epidural a therapy in which steroid is injected into the epidural space of the spine to relieve the pain of disc disease

Summer Heat conditions commonly occurring in the summer months in ancient times. They can vary from heat stroke to food poisoning since there was no refrigeration in antiquity.

sympathetic nervous system the part of the autonomic nervous system that is activated with stress. It gears the body for "fight or flight."

synergistic the mutually enhancing therapeutic effect of combining therapies such as drugs or herbs

Taoism the philosophy prevalent in China and influencing TCM. It purports that there is an order to the universe, the tao, which is maintained by the balance of dualistic forces. Taoists believe that illness begins with an imbalance of these forces.

T-cell cells made by the thymus gland for fighting infection

TCM traditional Chinese medicine

tendonitis an inflammation of tendons

tetanus a severe, life-threatening disease caused by the Clostridium tetanii toxin

thromboxane a substance produced by platelets that causes vaso-constriction and causes platelets to adhere to each other. It counterbalances the effects of prostacyclin.

titrate a method of determining the correct dosage of a therapy by increasing it stepwise until the desired effect is reached

tonification the therapeutic principle of restoring a weakened function or depleted bodily substance

tonify to replenish a depleted substance when it is deficient in order to restore function

toxic foods foods considered by TCM to have a toxic effect on the body, resulting in heat or inflammation

tumor necrosis factor a cytokine that promotes inflammation

uroshiol an allergenic substance present in poison oak and in mango skin

varicose ulcer a skin ulcer as a complication of varicose veins

varicose veins a condition in which the circulation of venous blood in the leg is poor, and the blood backs up and pools in the leg veins because of incompetent leg vein valves

vasectomy the male sterilization procedure in which the vas def-erens is severed

vasodilators drugs or herbs that act by relaxing the smooth muscles of blood vessel walls to dilate the blood vessel

vertigo the symptom of spinning experienced by patients with either an inner ear condition or an insufficient blood supply to the brain as a forewarning of a stroke

wood ear a naturally occurring fungus, used in Chinese cooking, that has an anticlotting property

Wet fluid overretention or overproduction

Wet-Heat a bodily immune response leading to inflammation

References

Alpha-Tocopherol, Beta Carotene Cancer Prevention Study Group. 1994. The effect of vitamin E and beta carotene on the incidence of lung cancer and other cancers in male smokers. *New Eng JM* 330:1029–34.

Astragalus membranaceus. 2003. Monograph. *Alternative Medicine Review* Feb.

Bensky, D. 1990. *Chinese herbal medicine formulas & strategies.* Comp. and trans. R. Barolet. Seattle, WA: Eastland Press.

———. 1987. *A Chinese herbal medicine materia medica.* Comp. and trans. Gamble, A. Seattle, WA: Eastland Press.

Bensoussan, A., N. J. Talley, M. Hing, R. Menzies, A. Guo, and M. Ngu. 1998. Treatment of irritable bowel syndrome with Chinese herbal medicine. *JAMA* 280:1585–1589.

Bertagnolli, M., et al. 2006. Celecoxib for the prevention of sporadic colorectal adenomas. *New Eng JM* 355:873–884.

Brashear, A., et al. 2002. Intramuscular injection of botulinum toxin for the treatment of wrist and finger spasticity after a stroke. *New Eng JM* 347:395–400.

Bresalier, R, et al. 2005. Cardiovascular events associated with rofecoxib in a colorectal adenoma chemoprevention trial. *New Eng JM* 352:1092–1102.

Buffon, A., et al. 2002. Widespread coronary inflammation in unstable angina. *New Eng JM* 347:6–12.

Cameron, B. 2004. Pharmacogenomics could replace 'trial and error' with science from the human genome. St. Jude Children's Research Hospital public release. www.stjude.org.

Cassidy, Claire M. 2002. *Contemporary Chinese medicine and acupuncture.* Philadelphia: Churchill Livingstone.

Cavallari, L., et al. 2006. Sex difference in the antiplatelet effect of aspirin in patients with stroke. *Ann Pharmacother* 405:812–7.

Chen, J., and N. Wang. 1988. *Acupuncture case histories from China.* Seattle, WA: Eastland Press.

Chilton, F. 2006. *Inflammation nation.* New York: Fireside.

Chinese acupuncture and moxibustion. 1993. Beijing: Foreign Language Press.

Chusid, J., and J. Mc Donald. 1958. *Correlative neuroanatomy and functional neurology,* Los Altos, CA: Lange Publications.

Cooper, D. A., A. L. Eldridge, and J. D. Peters. 1999. Dietary carotenoids and lung cancer: a review of recent research. *Nutr Rev* 57:133–45.

Davis, S., et al. 2001. The effects of Chinese medicinal herbs on postmenopausal vasomotor symptoms of Australian women: A randomised controlled trial. *Medical Journal of Australia* 174:68–71.

Dedier, J., et al. 2002. Nonnarcotic analgesic use and the risk of hypertension in US women. *Hypertension* 40:604–8.

Ellis, A., N. Wiseman, and K. Boss. 1989. *Grasping the wind.* Brookline, MA: Paradigm Publications.

Fadiman, A. 1997. *The spirit catches you and you fall down*. New York: Farrar, Straus and Giroux.

Falcone, M., et al. 1998. B Lymphocytes are crucial antigen-presenting cells in the pathogenic autoimmune response to gad 65 antigen in nonobese diabetic mice. *J of Immunology* 161:1163–68.

Ganong, W. 2003. *Review of medical physiology*. New York: McGraw Hill.

Gorman, C., and A. Park. 2002. A new science of headaches. *Time* October 7.

Grady-Weliky, T. 2003. Premenstrual dysphoric disorder. *New Eng JM* 348:433–435.

Gray, H. 1959. *Anatomy of the human body*. Philadelphia: Lea & Ferbiger.

Gunn, C. 1997. *Treatment of chronic pain*. New York: Churchill Livingstone.

———. 1989. *Treating myofascial pain*. Seattle, WA: University of Washington.

Hammerschmidt, D. 1980. Szechwan Purpura. *New Eng JM* 302:1191–93.

Helms, J. 1995. *Acupuncture energetics: A clinical approach for physicians*. Berkeley, CA: Medical Acupuncture Publishers.

Hotchkiss, R., and I. Karl. 2003. The pathophysiology and treatment of sepsis. *New Eng JM* 348.

Hsu, H. 1993a. *Chinese herb medicine and therapy*. Los Angeles, CA: Oriental Healing Arts Institute.

———. 1993b. *For women only: Chinese herbal formulas*. Los Angeles, CA: Oriental Healing Arts Institute.

Jiang, H., and L. Chess. 2006. Regulation of immune responses by T-Cells *New Eng JM* 354:1166–1176.

Joos, S., C. Schott, H. Zuo, V. Daniel, and E. Martin. 2000. Immunomodulatory effects of acupuncture in the treatment of allergic asthma: A randomized controlled study. *J Altern Complement Med* 6:519–525.

Kendall, D. 2002. *Dao of Chinese medicine: Understanding an ancient healing art.* Hong Kong: Oxford University Press (China) Ltd.

Klinger, H. C., et al. 2000. Use of peripheral neuromodulation of s3 region for treatment of detrusor overactivity: A urodynamic–based study. *Urology* 56:766–71.

Kurz, A., et al. 1996. Perioperative normothermia to reduce the incidence of surgical wound infection and shorten hospitalization. *New Eng JM* 334:1209–1216.

Lu, H. 1999. *Chinese natural cures.* New York: Black Dog & Leventhal.

Lyons, A., and R. Petrucelli II. 1987. *Medicine: An illustrated history.* New York: Harry N. Abrams, Inc.

Mah, A. 2000. *Watching the tree: A Chinese daughter reflects on happiness, traditions, and spiritual wisdom.* New York: Random House.

Mc Guire, E. 1983. Treatment of motor and sensory detrusor instability by electrical stimulation. *J Urol* 129:78–9.

Micklefield, G., et al. 1999. Effects of ginger on gastroduodenal motility. *Int J Clin Pharmacol Ther* 7:341–46.

Munglani, R., S. M. Harrison, G. D. Smith, C. Bountra, P. J. Birch, P. J. Elliot, and S. P. Hung. 1996. Neuropeptide changes persist in spinal cord despite resolving hyperalgesia mononeuropahy. *Brain Res* Dec 16:(1–2).

Naeser, Margaret. 1996. Research with acupuncture and laser acupuncture in the treatment of arm/leg paralysis and hand paresis in stroke. Lecture given at a symposium of the American Academy of Medical Acupuncture, San Francisco, June 6.

National Center for Biotechnology Information. 2004. One size does not fit all: The promise of pharmacogenomics. Mar 31 www.ncbi.nlm.nih.gov/About/primer/pharm.html.

Netter, F. 1989. *Atlas of human anatomy*. West Caldwell, NJ: Novartis.

Nissen, S., and Wolski, K. 2007. Effect of Rosiglitazone on the risk of myocardial infarction and death from cardiovascular causes. *New Eng JM* 356: 2457–70.

Nortier, J., et al. 2000. Urothelial carcinoma associated with the use of a Chinese herb (Aristolochia fangchi). *New Eng JM* 342:1686–92.

Nurse, Sir Paul. 2004. Interview by Charlie Rose, *Charlie Rose Show*, PBS December 20.

O'Connor, J. 1981. *Acupuncture: A comprehensive text*. Trans. D. Bensky. Chicago: Eastland Press.

Osborne, R. 1992. *Philosophy for beginners*. New York: Writers and Readers Publishing.

Paul, I. 2004. Dextromethorphan, Diphenhydramine ineffective for childhood cough. *Pediatrics* 114:83–90.

Perricone, N. 2004. *Perricone promise*. New York: Warner Books.

Pitchford,P. 1993. *Healing with whole foods: Oriental traditions and modern nutrition*. Berkeley, CA: North Atlantic Books.

Pharaoh's Obelisk. 1994. Secrets of Lost Empires II. *Nova*. PBS.

Porter, R. 1997. *Medicine: A history of healing: ancient traditions to modern practices*. East Sussex, U. K.: Ivy Press.

Practical Ear Needling Therapy. 1997. Hong Kong: Medicine and Health Publishing Co.

Ratner, R. 2005. Therapeutic role of incretin mimetics. *Medscape Diabetes & Endocrinology* 7:1–6. www.medscape.com.

Reid, D. 1996. *Traditional Chinese medicine.* Boston, MA: Shambala.

Schwartz, Cheryl. 1996. *Four Paws, Five Directions.* Berkeley, CA: Celestial Arts.

Solomon, S., et al. 2005. Cardiovascular risk associated with Celecoxib in a clinical trial for colorectal adenoma prevention. *New Eng JM* 352:1071–1080.

Song, T., 1986. *Atlas of tongues and lingual coatings in Chinese medicine.* Beijing: Joint Publication of People's Medical Publishing House.

Subotnick, S. 1991. *Sports & exercise injuries: Conventional, homeopathic, & alternative treatments.* Berkeley, CA: North Atlantic Books, Homeopathic Educational Services.

Unschuld, P. 1985. *Medicine in China: A history of ideas.* Berkeley, CA: University of California Press.

Vega, C., and L. Barclay. 2005. Artemether-Lumefantrine may be a superior combination for malaria treatment in resistant areas. *Medscape Medical News* April 25. 1–5.

Weiger, L. 1965. *Chinese characters: Their origin, etymology, history, classification and signification.* New York: Dover.

Wierzbicki, W., and K. Hagmeyer. 2000. Helicobacter pylori, Chlamydia pneumoniae, and Cytomegalovirus: Chronic infections and coronary heart disease. *Pharmacotherapy* 20:52–63.

Wiseman, N. 1996 *Fundamentals of Chinese medicine.* Trans. A. Ellis. Brookline, MA: Paradigm Publications.

Wong, J. 1999. *A manual of neuro-anatomical acupuncture.* Toronto, Canada: The Toronto Pain and Stress Clinic Inc.

Yehuda, R. 2002. Post-traumatic stress disorder. *New Eng JM* 346:108–114.

Yoder, K., et al. 2006. Child assessment of Dextromethorphan, Diphenhydramine, and placebo for nocturnal cough due to upper respiratory infection. *Clin Pediatr* (Phila) 45:663–40.

Yoo, T. 1988. *Koryo hand acupuncture.* Republic of Korea: Eum Yang Mek Jin Publishing Co.

Acknowledgments

The material for this book was gathered over many years, and many people deserve thanks for making the book possible. First are the faculty members of the American College of Traditional Chinese Medicine, who imparted their knowledge of traditional Chinese medicine to me. Then there are my lifelong teacher and mentor, Yat Ki Lai, and his wife, Shana Chan Lai, who have helped me to apply that knowledge to treat patients. I am also grateful for the patients whose stories of healing might help those readers who may recognize a similarity to their own afflictions.

For help with the actual writing, I thank my editors: Jane Ann Staw, Doris Ober, Rajinder Embody, and Lisa A. Smith. For moral support and encouragement, I am grateful to my friends and mentors at both the California Writers' Club and Bay Area Independent Publishers Association. Finally, I owe a debt of gratitude to my friends—Alice Au, Karen Chan, Fanida English, Joyce Devenny, Ed Hung, Diana Jung, Elena Krause, Nora Li, Angela Ng, Joyce Tang, and Lois VanderPol—who have endured reading my manuscript, some more than once, and giving me their suggestions. Whether heeded or not, I have pondered and weighed each one.

Herb Index

General Index

To Order this Book

You can either:
- Visit our website: www.balanceforhealthpublishing.com or
- Telephone: 1-800-852-4890 with your credit card information ready or
- Fax a copy of this page with your credit card information to 707-838-2220, or
- Mail this form with check payable to:

Rayve Productions
P. O. Box 726
Windsor, CA 95492-0726

Please send me

_____ copies of *Optimal Healing* at $19.95 each $ _____

_____ For 10 or more copies, discount rate is $15.95 each $ _____

Shipping $5.50 for first copy and $2.00 for each
additional copy $ _____

Shipping outside of the United States $15.00 for single book $ _____
For shipping rates of multiple books, please call 1-800-852-4890

Subtotal $ _____

California residents please add 7.75% sales tax of subtotal $ _____

Total $ _____

Please print

Name _____

Address _____

City _____ State _____ Zip _____

Telephone _____ E-Mail _____

☐ Check enclosed $ _____   Date _____

☐ Charge my Visa/MC/Discover/AMEX $ _____

Credit Card Number _____/_____/_____/_____

Expiration date _____/_____

Signature: _____

Returned checks: There is a $10.00 charge for any returned checks